Neil Solomon, M.D., Ph.D., is a specialist in the fields of endocrinology, metabolism, and allergy, and a nationally recognized authority on diet and weight control. A familiar figure to television viewers, Dr. Solomon also writes a nationally syndicated column that appears in more than 200 newspapers in the United States and Canada. His most popular other works include THE TRUTH ABOUT WEIGHT CONTROL and DR. SOLOMON'S MASTER PLAN FOR TOTAL BODY FITNESS AND MAINTENANCE.

Berkley books by Dr. Neil Solomon

DR. SOLOMON'S HIGH HEALTH DIET
AND EXERCISE PLAN

DR. SOLOMON'S PROVEN MASTER PLAN
FOR TOTAL BODY FITNESS AND MAINTENANCE

HOW TO MAKE CHOLESTEROL WORK FOR YOU

DOCTOR SOLOMON'S HIGH HEALTH DIET & EXERCISE PLAN

DR. NEIL SOLOMON

BERKLEY BOOKS, NEW YORK

This Berkley book contains the complete text of the original hardcover edition. It has been completely reset in a type face designed for easy reading, and was printed from new film.

DR. SOLOMON'S HIGH HEALTH DIET AND EXERCISE PLAN

A Berkley Book / published by arrangement with G. P. Putnam's Sons

PRINTING HISTORY
G. P. Putnam's Sons edition / June 1980
Berkley edition / March 1982

ISBN: 0-425-05086-6

A BERKLEY BOOK ® TM 757,375
Berkley Books are published by Berkley Publishing Corporation, 200 Madison Avenue, New York, New York 10016.
PRINTED IN THE UNITED STATES OF AMERICA

The author gratefully acknowledges permission to reprint from the following:

"Relation of Diet to High-Density-Lipoprotein Cholesterol in Middle-Aged Marathon Runners, Joggers, and Inactive Men," by G. Harley Hartung, Ph.D., John P. Foreyt, Ph.D., Robert E. Mitchell, Ph.D., Imogene Vlasek, M.Ed., and Antonio M. Gotto, Jr., M.D., Department of Medicine and Physical Medicine, Baylor College of Medicine, and The Methodist Hospital, Houston, Tx.

United Fresh Fruit and Vegetable Association, Alexandria, Virginia.

The United States Department of Agriculture Publications, Washington, D.C.

Fish Fat Content guide, Communications, Incorporated, San Antonio, Tx.

Margarine, Oil, and Dressing guide, *The Medical Letter*, New Rochelle, New York.

Kasch Pulse Recovery Test Protocol and Norms, Fred Kasch, Ph.D., San Diego, Ca.

Textbook of Work Physiology, by Per-Olaf Astrand, and Kaare Rodahl, Copyright © 1977 by McGraw-Hill Book Company, Inc.

Food Facts from Rutgers, Rutgers State University, New Jersey.

CONTENTS

INTRODUCTION

Today, there is a growing awareness that the food you eat affects your health and your whole life. Every day, exciting advances are being made in nutritional science. The work going forward in laboratories here and abroad shows that changes in your diet can actually lessen your risk of serious disease and increase your chances of enjoying more health for more years.

These findings are vital to your well-being—and to the well-being of your family and everyone close to you. In order to help you make them part of your everyday life, I have written the *High Health Diet and Exercise Plan*. In the pages of this book, I give you the programs that succeed with my patients. They are ones that you and every other reader can also have success with.

It is important for you to know why I feel such a great need to write this book and why I feel it essential to tell you how you can make a substance that you have heard a lot about recently, cholesterol, work *for* you rather than *against* you—as it unfortunately does for so many people.

It is common scientific knowledge that the overly rich diet people eat today—people in every part of this country and in other prosperous countries—is linked with serious diseases: heart disease, strokes, high blood pressure, certain cancers, diabetes, gallbladder disease, obesity. By far the most definite link is between this rich diet and America's number-one killer, cardiovascular disease in which cholesterol is a key factor.

There has been a great deal written about cholesterol in the past few years—all of it bad. We are now finding, however, that there has been an oversimplification and misunderstanding of what cholesterol is and what it does. You cannot generalize about cholesterol. Different kinds of cholesterol must be distinguished between, because they act in very different ways: one kind does good and another kind does harm. And researchers are now showing that your cholesterol balance can be improved by changing your diet.

Exercise, too, can have a healthful effect on your cholesterol balance. The right exercise increases the level of good cholesterol and decreases the bad. I am giving you the exercise routines that I give to my patients. The High Health Diet together with the Exercise Plan really do show you all the ways you can make your cholesterol work for you.

The High Health Diet and Exercise Plan is good for everyone—men and women, young and old, the whole family. And if you are trying to lose some weight, the diet has built-in, low-calorie benefits—so you can combine it with routines in the Exercise Plan for excellent results.

I particularly want to emphasize one thing: prevention. To protect yourself against the big killers like heart disease, prevention must be your strategy; because in spite of the great strides that science has made, we do not yet have a cure for many killer diseases. There is much that doctors can do to alleviate them or delay their worst results, but the only way to play it really safe is prevention. You must do the things that can prevent these killers. That means the correct kind of diet and exercise.

The sooner you begin, the more benefits you will gain. But you will have improvement at any age—whether you are sixty-seven or twenty-three. Whatever your age, whatever shape you are in, start right away. Be high on health for the rest of your life!

1

High Health and Cholesterol

Cholesterol meant nothing to most people until ten or fifteen years ago. But by now it has become a household word from coast to coast. You can't turn on your TV or open your paper without being told that cholesterol can clog up your blood vessels and lead to a heart attack or a stroke.

However, cholesterol isn't quite the villain it has been made out to be. We have known all along that it has many essential functions in the body. And although it can indeed be a big factor in hardening of the arteries (atherosclerosis), the latest research shows that there is actually a good kind of blood cholesterol as well as a bad kind.

Before we get to that, though, let's first have a quick look at some of the basics about cholesterol. First . . .

JUST WHAT IS CHOLESTEROL?

Cholesterol is a pearly white, tasteless, odorless, crystalline substance—one of the many kinds of *sterols,* waxy alcohols which in turn belong to a large chemical class called lipids. The fats and oils you are familiar with in everyday life are also lipids. Cholesterol is sometimes casually referred to as one of the blood fats, but this is not scientifically correct.

It is the most common sterol in animals, but with only a few exceptions, cholesterol does not occur in plants. They have their own kinds of sterols, like phytosterol and sitosterol. Some sterols are found in both animals and plants—ergosterol, for instance. (You have ergosterol in your skin, and under the sun's radiation it changes to vitamin D, which protects against rickets. That is why a certain amount of sunshine was so important for children in the days when we didn't have vitamin-D supplements in milk and other foods.)

WHAT IS CHOLESTEROL FOR?

Cholesterol does many very important things in the body. It is a key part of brain tissue. It goes into the sheaths that protect nerve fibers. You need cholesterol for your sex hormones (and most of your other hormones as well), for the membranes of all your cells, for your skin, for many other vital body compounds. It plays an important role in the body's metabolism. It is an essential part of bile, without which you could not digest fat. In other words, if you did not have cholesterol you could not live. Not that you need a great deal of it. By weight, you are about three-tenths of 1 percent cholesterol. If you are a woman and weigh 120 pounds, you have 5 or 6 ounces of cholesterol throughout your body. If you are a man and weigh 150 pounds, you have 7 or 8 ounces.

WHERE DOES IT COME FROM?

Most of your cholesterol is made by your own body. Practically any body tissue can manufacture it, but the main cholesterol-producing unit is the liver. It can make as much as 2 grams a day. You also get some cholesterol in the food you eat.

CHOLESTEROL CHEMISTRY

Cholesterol is made up of carbon, hydrogen, and oxygen—the chemical trio that is basic to all life. There are thousands of fantastically complicated ways in which these three elements combine to make different substances. In the case of cholesterol, the formula is C27 H45 OH. This means that the cholesterol molecule has 27 carbon atoms plus 45 hydrogen atoms (arranged in several six-sided rings) plus a special oxygen-hydrogen unit called a hydroxyl. The hydroxyl is connected to a radical. A radical, in chemistry, is a group of atoms that remains stable even if the molecule is undergoing changes. It is a sort of anchorman—a good, reliable fellow.

WHEN DID WE FIND OUT ABOUT CHOLESTEROL?

Cholesterol was discovered over a century and a half ago—in 1812, to be exact—when it was isolated from gallstones. That is how it got its name ("*cholē*" means gall or bile in Greek).

Another important discovery came almost exactly a hundred years later, in 1913, when a Russian scientist, N. N. Anitschow, found that he could cause atherosclerosis in rabbits by feeding them large quantities of cholesterol. This touched off a spate of research, but it did not change the prevailing medical view, which held that atherosclerosis and heart disease were simply the inevitable accompaniment of old age.

Here is what a very well-known physician, Dr. Logan Clendening, wrote in 1927: "What, after all, are those mysterious things—high blood pressure and hardening of the arteries? Merely the process of growing old. That and nothing more. Why all the pother?"

Well, we know now that hardening of the arteries and high blood pressure (hypertension) are not merely part of growing old. Much of the new understanding came during and just after World War II. Researchers noticed how low-fat diets imposed in a number of European countries by the shortage of meat and other rich foods were followed by a decrease in heart disease.

Then in the 1950s and 1960s, studies covering a range of countries showed two very important things:

1. There is a definite link between heart disease and blood cholesterol.

2. Blood cholesterol tends to be high when the diet has a lot of fat (specifically, animal fat) and cholesterol in it.

CHOLESTEROL AND LIPOPROTEINS

As I mentioned earlier, we have now discovered that we can't think of cholesterol just as one simple thing. It is important to know what *kind* of cholesterol it is.

Here is what goes on. The blood carries a continuous two-way flow of cholesterol and other lipids between the liver, the intestines, and other tissues of the body where they are used or stored or excreted. But the blood lipids do not travel all by themselves. They are moved around in tiny packets called lipoproteins, which are made up of lipids and protein. It is as if cholesterol and the other lipids were riding piggyback on the protein. The lipids are picked up and deposited through intricate electronic and chemical processes at their various points of departure and arrival.

There are two main kinds of lipoproteins—high-density lipoprotein, or HDL for short, and low-density lipoprotein, LDL for short.

HDL is about half protein, and has smaller amounts of cholesterol and a lipid called phospholipid in addition to a small quantity of triglyceride (a triglyceride, made up of three fatty acids and one molecule of glycerol, is the most common kind of fat). HDL accounts for about 20 to 25 percent of the total amount of cholesterol in the blood.

LDL has more than twice as much cholesterol as HDL and only half as much protein. With some exceptions, most of the blood's cholesterol is carried in the LDL form—anywhere from a half to two-thirds or more.

There are three other lipoproteins that I will mention briefly.

One is the very-low-density lipoprotein (VLDL) which contains a large amount of triglyceride.

Another is a rare type called intermediate-low-density lipoprotein (ILDL) which seems to be a transitional form between VLDL and LDL.

And the third is chylomicrons, which are made up almost entirely of phospholipid.

None of these three contain a significant amount of cholesterol.

GOOD GUYS-BAD GUYS

HDL is the good guy. *The more HDL you have, the less your heart risk. If your total cholesterol is high because you have a lot of HDL, count yourself lucky.*

LDL is the bad guy. *The more low-density lipoprotein you have, the greater your risk. And if your total cholesterol is high because you have a lot of LDL, that is cause for concern.*

We start off life with about half of our cholesterol in the form of HDL. As we grow up and get into the habit of eating too many rich foods, the proportion of HDL drops to about a quarter.

Interestingly enough, animals that have no heart attacks to speak of, like dogs and cats and minks, have about three-quarters of their blood cholesterol in HDL. On the other hand, animals whose heart disorders are similar to human's, such as pigs and rabbits, have high levels of LDL.

Eskimos have high cholesterol levels, but virtually no heart attacks because their HDL is high and their LDL is low. And a Cincinnati study has identified some families with extremely high HDL readings whose members remain healthy into their eighties and nineties.

HOW DO HDL AND LDL WORK?

We do not know exactly how HDL does its good work. It may prevent the buildup of fats on the walls of blood vessels. It may also act as a scavenger, cleaning off cholesterol deposits and taking them to the liver where they are converted into bile acids and then excreted.

LDL's primary function, on the other hand, seems to be to carry cholesterol from the liver or the intestines to other parts of the body. It is when there is too much of this LDL in the bloodstream that there is trouble.

The mechanism of the atherosclerotic buildup in blood vessels is extremely complicated and not yet fully understood. It may start with a microscopic injury which promotes some excess cell growth. This in turn may accumulate cholesterol and other substances, like a river silting up where protrusions catch debris. In any case, the LDL and HDL in the blood play major roles—one harmful, the other helpful—in this process.

WHEN DOES ALL THIS START?

Much earlier than you may think. Even in the teens there are often some fatty streaks forming in the blood vessels. Later, by the late twenties or thirties, there may be a definite narrowing of the vessels as fatty, fibrous plaques appear. By age forty or so—in American men, at least—these plaques may begin to calcify.

WHEN DOES THIS BECOME REALLY DANGEROUS?

It is impossible to say precisely when the danger point is reached. But as a blood vessel narrows, there is an increasing chance of a blood clot blocking the channel completely. The clot may form locally, or be riding along in the bloodstream—and get caught in the narrow spot. When this happens in a coronary artery (one nourishing the heart), it is a heart attack—some of the heart muscle dies for lack of oxygen-carrying blood. If it happens in the brain, it is a stroke. It can also occur in other parts of the body, such as the kidney, with serious and perhaps fatal results.

MEASURING YOUR CHOLESTEROL

Until the new studies on HDL and LDL came along, it was thought that only the *total* amount of cholesterol in your blood mattered. The theory went, the more you had, the greater your risk of heart disease or stroke. If you were told to watch your cholesterol because it was, say, 260 (meaning 260 milligrams per 100 milliliters), that 260 figure mentioned by the doctor was the total figure. Now many doctors feel you should have a more detailed analysis of your blood cholesterol so you know how you really stand. In other words, you want to know how your HDL compares to your LDL. You want to know your *cholesterol balance*.

One way of doing this is to measure HDL and total cholesterol. The difference between them corresponds to the LDL level.

WHAT SHOULD YOUR CHOLESTEROL BE?

Let's start with HDL. The average HDL figure for American men is 45—meaning, 45 milligrams per 100 milliliters. The average for women is a good bit higher: 55. This is clearly one reason women have fewer heart attacks than do men.

For a man, 55 would generally be a good reading (there have been HDL levels as high as 125). On the other hand, if HDL is down to something like 35, that suggests a definitely increased risk unless LDL is also quite low.

How about total cholesterol? Sometimes up to 250 is described as a "normal" range for an American man. But this is likely to be too high for good health. As a rule, the lower the total cholesterol level, the better. In populations where the "normal" level is around 150 there are virtually no heart attacks.

In any case, the really important thing is the *proportion* that goes into HDL and LDL. Dr. William Castelli, one of the main researchers in the famous Framingham heart study (which has been following several thousand people for some three decades), says a good way to check this ratio is to compare the total to the HDL: total cholesterol/HDL cholesterol.

If the ratio is 5 to 1 (in other words if the total cholesterol is five times HDL), that would be an average risk in the United States, but, as I said, one that is too high. A desirable ratio would be 3.5 to 1, or less. On the other hand, a ratio of 10 to 1 would be double the standard risk.

Dr. Castelli says that the total cholesterol figure by itself is still useful for measuring risk among younger people, but is of decreasing value with age, and is not at all useful once you are past fifty.

However, the total cholesterol figure is still used by many doctors as a useful index. Since it appears in medical studies going back several decades, researchers will have to keep using it for purposes of comparison. So the new measurements refine and correct the old, single reading rather than replacing it entirely.

WHAT ABOUT TRIGLYCERIDES—ARE THEY HARMFUL?

Excessive levels of triglyceride in the blood can be harmful too. They may be due to obesity or excess consumption of sugar, in which case they can be reduced by losing weight and cutting sugar consumption. Serious cases of high blood triglycerides are not common. They are likely to be hereditary and require special dietary treatment.

BOOSTING YOUR HDL, LOWERING YOUR LDL

Now you want to know what you can do about your cholesterol to minimize your chances of heart trouble. Diet is very important. And so is exercise. And there are other factors too. More about all this in the following chapters.

etable protein for at least some of it makes a lot of health sense. Americans eat much more protein than they need, and over two-thirds of it is of animal origin. In populations where heart disease is rare, protein consumption is much lower and almost all of it is from vegetable sources.

There is an additional and very interesting point. A number of experts feel that earliest man was primarily vegetarian—that in the beginning, we ate plant food rather than meat. Heavy meat consumption may be going against nature and overloading the metabolism that was developed by a long evolutionary process.

So a greater emphasis on vegetables in general—and that includes grains, legumes, nuts, and seeds—is a wise move. And fruits too, of course. This is one of the main principles of the High Health Diet.

SOY

There is growing evidence that soybeans are very healthful. Let me cite two recent medical reports.*

Dr. C. R. Sartori and colleagues in Milan, Italy, have found in their experiments that soy can lower total cholesterol very markedly. They worked with twenty patients who had high total cholesterol levels and who were already on a standard low-fat diet. What Dr. Sartori did was remove the animal protein and replace it with soybean textured protein. Otherwise the diet remain unchanged.

In three weeks, the soy diet resulted in a 21 percent decrease in the total cholesterol level, and a 23 percent decrease in LDL cholesterol—a striking result. Dr. Sartori repeated the test successfully with another, smaller group of patients. He also found that the soy had its beneficial effect even when a rather large amount of cholesterol was added to the diet—500 milligrams

*G. Harley Hartung, Ph.D., John P. Foreyt, Ph.D., Robert E. Mitchell, Ph.D., Imogene Vlasek, M.Ed., and Antonio M. Gotto, Jr., M.D., "Relation of Diet to High-Density-Lipoprotein Cholesterol in Middle-Aged Marathon Runners, Joggers, and Inactive Men."

daily, the amount you would get in two egg yolks.

Earlier studies had also shown that substituting soy protein for meat protein lowered blood cholesterol. However, experts had thought it could simply have been because soybean doesn't have the saturated fat and cholesterol that meat does.

But Dr. Sartori isolated the effect of the soy by keeping the saturated fat and cholesterol in the first soy diet the same as in the non-soy diet (and there was actually *more* cholesterol in the second soy diet). His conclusion: Soy protein, *as such,* has a cholesterol-lowering effect compared to meat protein. (An extra plus was that the patients liked the appearance and taste of the meals with soy dishes).

Another experiment with similar results has been done by Dr. K. K. Carroll and colleagues of the University of Western Ontario in London, Ontario. This time the volunteers were young, healthy women with normal cholesterol levels. First they ate an average diet with mixed protein, and then switched to one in which the animal protein was replaced by soy-textured protein and soy milk. The saturated fat and cholesterol content was kept essentially the same.

Here again, the total cholesterol level in the blood was lowered. The shift was not so marked as in the tests done by Dr. Sartori. But this is not surprising as the women in the Canadian tests had normal cholesterol levels to begin with, whereas the Italian patients had high levels.

MILK

Milk, we know, is an excellent food. It is true that there has been concern about the fat in whole milk—and that is why skim milk is preferable. But new studies indicate that milk of any kind can actually lower the cholesterol level in your blood.

Two British researchers, J. Marks and A. N. Howard of Cambridge, England, have had this result with a number of experiments. Even whole milk worked, despite its saturated fat, although skim milk was more effective. A Danish researcher has suggested that lactose, the milk sugar, may be what causes the cholesterol drop. But the British experts don't think this can be the whole story. They have obtained a 7 percent reduction using lactose alone—but a 15 percent reduction using skim milk.

Dr. George V. Mann, of Vanderbilt University in Tennessee, has also found that milk lowers serum cholesterol levels, perhaps by preventing its buildup in the blood. He thinks this is due to a specific ingredient which he calls M.F. (Milk Factor). Certain kinds of processing may remove M.F., he notes, as cholesterol levels do increase after eating butter.

YOGURT

Dr. Mann has found that yogurt is more effective than milk in lowering cholesterol. He discovered the virtues of yogurt by chance while doing some dietary experiments with the Masai warriors in Africa. The Masai are remarkably healthy and virtually immune to heart disease. The mainstay of their diet happens to be yogurt, although they have a meat binge once a week—and drink straight blood from time to time. Their total blood cholesterol is extremely low—about 135 compared to the American male average of well over 200.

Dr. Mann's experiments, which originally concentrated on a group of food additives called surfactants, involved the offering of free yogurt to a group of 24 young Masai warriors who volunteered for the test. The free meal was a big drawing card. The warriors came back for more, and ended up daily consuming 2 gallons of yogurt apiece. This was whole-milk yogurt, mind you, and they did, of course, put on weight.

But despite the weight gain, and the large intake of dietary cholesterol and saturated fat, their serum cholesterol levels went down—from their already very low level. The more yogurt they ate, the lower their blood cholesterol fell.

Dr. Mann concluded that there was something in the yogurt that blocked cholesterol production in the liver—and more than offset the big increase in dietary cholesterol. He repeated his experiment with doctors and scientists back at Vanderbilt, and achieved cholesterol reductions of up to a third. I am not suggesting that you imitate the Masai and eat 2 gallons of yogurt a day, but it certainly is a good idea to include yogurt regularly in your diet.

FISH

Fish has been neglected in the American diet, and that is a great pity. Fish is a first-rate source of protein and has an extremely healthful balance of fats. The fat content varies from species to species, and some fish are quite fatty, but fish oils are predominantly unsaturated—either polyunsaturated or monounsaturated and the saturated-fat content is invariably low.

FIBER

You have probably been hearing lots about fiber recently. To believe some people, it is the cure-all to end all cure-alls. But, discounting these excessive claims, there is no doubt that fiber is an important and neglected part of a healthful diet—especially certain kinds of fiber. There are many different kinds of fiber. And there is still a great deal that we do not know about the effect of all of them in our diet.

You may ask, just what do we mean by "fiber" in general? It can be defined as the structural parts of fruit, stems, flowers, seeds, leaves, and roots of different plants—little, if any, of which is absorbed. One important kind of fiber is cellulose, which is found in the cell walls of plants. Another fiber group includes substances like pectin (also found in the cell walls), mucilages (from the seeds), and gums (from the plant's surface). A third group is made up of woody substances called lignins.

It has been said that fiber *in general* lowers cholesterol levels. But the most careful researchers narrow this down to certain kinds of fiber.

One of these is *pectin*, which is found abundantly in fruits such as apples and oranges, and which is the substance that makes jelly gel.

Certain *gums* are also effective, such as guar (from a bean) and locust-bean gum.

Rolled oats, (more particularly the hulls) also lower cholesterol.

Soybean hulls have been found to lower total cholesterol.

On the other hand, Dr. A. Stewart Truswell, a leading British authority, reports that wheat fiber is ineffective and that the same goes for cellulose except in very large quantities. Dr. Hans Fisher of Rutgers also advises that widely advertised cellulose and wheat bran do not lower cholesterol.

ALCOHOL

One finding in recent studies came as a pleasant surprise to many people. Moderate drinking actually lowers LDL and raises HDL.

One study found that someone who drank 5 to 6 ounces of alcohol a week—the equivalent of 1 cocktail or 2 modest glasses of wine a day—had about 10 percent more HDL and less LDL than teetotalers.

Just how this occurs is not clear. It may be that a certain level of alcohol slows the absorption of LDL by cells. Or perhaps the primary factor is that the alcohol raises the HDL level, and this in turn affects the LDL.

None of this, of course, should encourage excessive drinking, which can damage the heart as well as wreak a great deal of other havoc throughout the mind and body. But it does indicate that *moderate* drinking can be not only pleasant but healthful.

Alcoholic beverages should be eliminated from the diet by persons under twenty-one years of age.

3

The High Health Diet Guidelines: Fats, Carbohydrates, Protein

I said earlier that if you are eating anything like the average American diet you should cut down your consumption of fat. You may wonder: Is there a minimum that you should get? The answer to that is yes—but it is a very small amount.

There is one "fatty acid" you must have in your diet because your body needs it but cannot make it. It is called linoleic acid. Eliminating it from the diet causes skin troubles and stunts growth. It is plentiful in vegetable oils like safflower, soybean, corn and cottonseed. To get your necessary quota of linoleic acid, all you have to do is to have 1 or 2 percent of your calories in fat containing it. However, it's better to have somewhat more to offset the saturated fat that you get in your food. Linoleic acid is a polyunsaturate.

There is one other essential function of dietary fat, and that is to bring you certain vitamins—the so-called fat-soluble vitamins: A, D, E, and K. But here again only a minute amount of fat is involved.

Many people like fat for the taste and texture it provides in food. Pure fat actually has no taste at all, but it is good at retaining flavors. Also, it gives you a feeling of satiety by slowing the emptying of the stomach.

So do not feel that you have to go on some very austere and spartan regime. The High Health Diet is not that at all. You will find it delicious and satisfying as well as healthful. The point I want to emphasize here is that the amount of fat you actually need in your diet is very small.

SATURATED/UNSATURATED

A fatty acid is a chain of oxygen, hydrogen, and carbon. If one, two or three of these chains are hitched to a molecule of glycerine, you have a fatty acid.

When a fatty acid has as much hydrogen as it can hold, in other words when there is a hydrogen atom occupying each available space, we say it is *saturated*. It looks like this:

```
 H H H H H H H H H H H H H H H H H
 | | | | | | | | | | | | | | | | |
HC-C-C-C-C-C-C-C-C-C-C-C-C-C-C-C-C-COOH
 | | | | | | | | | | | | | | | | |
 H H H H H H H H H H H H H H H H H
```

When two spaces are empty (the spaces come in pairs), the fatty acid is *monounsaturated*. Meaning that it has *one* (mono) pair of empty spaces like this:

```
 H H H H H H H H H   H H H H H H H H
 | | | | | | | | |   | | | | | | | |
HC-C-C-C-C-C-C-C-C = C-C-C-C-C-C-C-C-COOH
 | | | | | | | |       | | | | | | |
 H H H H H H H H       H H H H H H H
```

When there are four, six, eight or more unoccupied places, the fatty acid is *polyunsaturated* ("poly" is from the Greek word for "many"). Like:

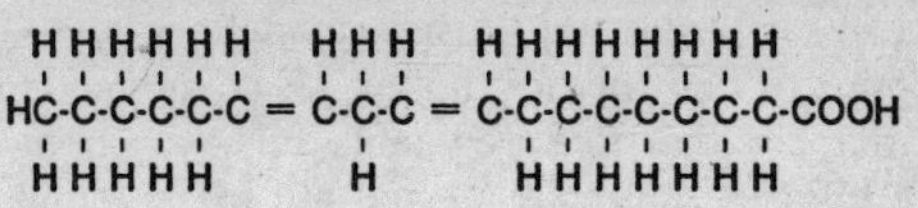

Food fats contain varying mixtures of all three kinds of fatty acids. When we talk about saturated fats, what we really mean is fats with a high proportion of saturated fatty acids. Animal fat is in this category. A monounsaturated fat—such as olive oil—has a lot of monounsaturated fatty acids. A polyunsaturated fat has a lot of polyunsaturated fatty acids. All vegetable oils except coconut and palm are in this group.

Saturated fats are generally solid at room temperature. You have probably noticed how beef fat gets hard when it isn't warm. That is because it is very saturated. On the other hand, chicken fat is less saturated and you may have noticed that it does not harden the way beef fat does, even if refrigerated. Fish fat is even more polyunsaturated.

In commercial processing, hydrogen may be added to fats and oils to harden them. If you see "hydrogenated" on the label, that means the maximum amount of hydrogen that the fat will hold has been added. "Partially hydrogenated" means there is still room for extra hydrogen.

FAT AND BLOOD CHOLESTEROL

As we noted before, eating a lot of saturated fat has a bad effect on your blood cholesterol as it tends to raise the LDL. On the other hand, polyunsaturated fat tends to lower LDL. Monounsaturated fat does not seem to affect the cholesterol balance one way or the other.

All this does not mean that you should cut out saturated fat entirely, or go on a polyunsaturated binge. Medical authorities, among them the American Heart Association, think that a good balance consists of about a third of your fat calories in the monounsaturated form, not more than a third in the saturated form, and at least a third in the polyunsaturated form.

You can easily stay within these guidelines by reducing your consumption of rich cheeses, butter, ice cream, and fatty meats. Also remember that two vegetable oils—coconut and palm oil—are high in saturated fat and are often found in bakery products and other processed foods.

As I said before, vegetable oils are excellent sources of polyunsaturates. The margarines that you find in little tubs are also good. Stick margarine is generally preferable to butter but is not so good as tub margarine because it has been partially hydrogenated.

Olive oil and peanut oil have a great deal of monounsaturated fat.

FAT AND DIETARY CHOLESTEROL

A good many people do not understand that saturated fat and dietary cholesterol are two distinct things. Some foods that are high in saturated fat also happen to be high in cholesterol, but very often the levels of the two ingredients will be quite different. For instance, organ meats such as brains and liver are very high in cholesterol content but have very little saturated fat. Beef has a lot of saturated fat and a moderate amount of cholesterol. Coconut oil has no cholesterol at all but has a lot of saturated fat. Chicken has a moderate amount of saturated fat and is low in cholesterol. Fish is low in both.

Vegetables, fruits, and grains have no cholesterol at all—and with just a few exceptions no saturated fat to speak of.

CARBOHYDRATES

Carbohydrates, the sugars and starches, are our chief source of energy. The main carbohydrate foods are the vegetable, fruit and grain group. Carbohydrates come in all chemical shapes and sizes of various complexity, but the basic unit is always carbon plus H_2O. They are all broken down into very simple sugars in digestion, the most important being glucose, which fuels the whole body and is the only kind of energy the brain and the central nervous system can use.

Since early in this century, the proportion of calories that Americans get from carbohydrates has been going down—from about 60 percent to the present 46 percent. Of this smaller amount, the proportion of *refined* carbohydrates—sugar and white starch—has increased drastically. During the same period, coronary heart disease has zoomed from a medical rarity to the nation's leading killer. In countries where heart disease is rare, people get anywhere from 65 to 85 percent of their calories from carbohydrate.

So you can see that getting more of the healthful complex carbohydrates in vegetables, grains and fruits, as we do in the High Health Diet, makes good sense.

IS CARBOHYDRATE FATTENING?

Some people mistakenly think that foods rich in carbohydrates are fattening. They're not unless they're cakes, pies and junk food. Natural carbohydrates like fruits and vegetables yield 4 calories per gram—just like protein, and less than half what fat does. Besides having lots of important vitamins and minerals, natural carbohydrate-rich foods are also our main source of fiber, which has no calories at all.

SUGARS AND SUGARS

When we think of "sugar" as fattening, we are thinking of *refined* sugar (generally sucrose)—which is a very concentrated form of calories. It is so easy to slip two or three teaspoons of sugar into a cup of coffee and gobble up a sugar doughnut. To get the same amount of sugar in its natural complete form, you would have to eat 2 or 3 pounds of apples or beets.

I would like to make three medical points about refined

sugar. One, it is bad for your teeth—it is the favorite meal of the bacteria that produce the acid which destroys the enamel. (The main thing you should avoid is frequent sweet snacks throughout the day.)

Second, refined sugar provides energy and nothing else—no vitamins or minerals. It is "empty calories."

Third, some researchers, like Dr. Yudkin in England, believe that high sucrose consumption is a factor in heart disease. However, most experts feel that this case has not yet been proven. In any event, there are many excellent reasons to cut down on refined sugar consumption.

FIBER: SPECIAL CARBOHYDRATES

During the last few years there has been an upsurge of interest in dietary fiber. The pioneers in this field were Dr. Dennis Burkitt and other English researchers. They were struck by the fact that primitive peoples in Africa seemed virtually free of "diseases of civilization"—like coronary heart disease, cancer, appendicitis, and diverticulitis (hernia-like pouches protruding from the intestine). They noted that these peoples had much more roughage in their diet than did Westerners.

The theory they proposed was this: there seemed to be some cause-and-effect link between the shift to a low-fiber diet and the appearance of the diseases of civilization.

IS FIBER A CURE-ALL?

Some people have latched on to this hypothesis and promoted fiber as a miracle food. Add it to your diet, they say, and you'll live to be a hundred. I do not go along with these exaggerated claims, but I do think we should have more fiber in our diet.

The two points on which there is general medical agreement are that fiber is effective against constipation, and may often be the best way to prevent or treat diverticulitis. The relation between fiber and heart disease or intestinal cancer requires a great deal more research.

In any case, fiber is a catch-all term for a host of substances, most of which are extremely complicated carbohydrates. As we noted in Chapter 2 we are finding that certain of these, like pectin and rolled oats, have a good effect on blood cholesterol.

Summing up, you can't go wrong with fiber if you simply increase the amount of fruit, vegetables, and grains in your diet.

PROTEIN

Protein is an essential part of your body, and it is an essential part of your diet. But it is not the magic ingredient that so many people think it is.

In your body, protein is the major structural component. It holds together your muscles, tendons, skin and other tissues. It is in your hormones, blood, bones, genes. It is part of every cell you have. There are thousands of different kinds of body protein, but they are all made up of various combinations of about 20 nitrogen compounds called amino acids.

Your body is not static. It is being torn down and rebuilt continuously. There is a certain amount of waste in this process—you lose protein in your sweat, urine, hair, nails and sloughed-off skin. Your body can make most of the amino acids it needs to build new protein, but there are eight that it cannot produce and which you must get in your food. They are called the essential amino acids.

How do you get them? Animal products are a good source because they provide the eight essential amino acids in an effective balance. This does not mean that they have to be red meat. Fish is excellent. So is poultry—and milk. White of egg is about the best you can get.

Also—and this is something that too many people fail to realize—vegetables and grains provide protein. One or two of the essential amino acids may be missing or in short supply, but this problem can easily be overcome by mixing different vegetable foods, or adding a little animal protein to the dish. That way you get a well-balanced package of essential amino acids. Some vegetable proteins are as effective as animal proteins—soy is a good example.

HOW MUCH PROTEIN DO YOU NEED?

Much less than you think. Unless you are on some very kooky diet, it is practically impossible to live in America and not get enough protein.

Let's look at some figures. The RDA (Recommended Dietary Allowance) is 46 grams for the average woman and 56 for the average man. You would get that from a pint of skim milk plus a small serving of fish or chicken plus a dish of rice and beans. And that is not even counting other protein sources, such as bread!

The RDA figure is not a bare minimum. It is higher than other estimates drawn up by nutrition authorities. For instance, the Food and Agricultural Organization's recommendation is 29 grams of protein per day for an adult woman.

What about those protein supplements you keep hearing about? Forget them, they are a waste of money. They may actually harm your body if taken in excess. For one thing, they can overload and damage your kidneys as you try to get rid of excess nitrogen that your system cannot use.

There is growing evidence that the high protein diet so many Americans think is healthful is not healthful at all. That is aside from the fact that so much of our protein comes with a lot of saturated fat.

But doesn't extra protein give you energy? Protein is indeed a source of energy, just as carbohydrate and fat are. But it is expensive, and not very efficient. The carbohydrate you get from vegetables, grains, and fruits are a much better energy source. Sports doctors and trainers now stress that even top athletes burning thousands of calories a day do not need extra protein. And that they are, in fact, better off without it.

How about children? As they are growing they do need a

good supply of protein. And children will get plenty of protein with the High Health Diet. So will pregnant women.

HIGH HEALTH FOODS

How do you carry out these recommendations in practice? What foods should you go in for? Which should you go easy on or even do without entirely?

First of all, put much more emphasis on *vegetables, fruit and grain*. They bring you the energy-giving carbohydrate you need in its most healthful form. They provide you with a whole range of vitamins and minerals. They help you cut down on your consumption of fat and get trim and stay trim. They help lower your total blood cholesterol.

Also, *the vegetable-grain family can give you very good protein*. Especially if you get a variety and mix grains with beans or peas. And we have seen earlier how the soybean in particular is not only a first-rate source of complete protein but also raises the good-guy kind of cholesterol, HDL.

• Good daily amounts: 6 servings of vegetables; 3 to 4 of fruit; 4 to 5 bread or other grain product.

Secondly, include *fish* regularly. It is such a good source of protein and polyunsaturated fat, and makes for a good cholesterol balance.

• Good daily amount: 5 ounces of fish, poultry or meat. This amount equals 35 grams of protein. The remaining protein is derived from milk, yogurt, eggs, and whole grain vegetables.

The most healthful diets in the world are predominantly vegetarian with a little animal protein added. The High Health Diet is one of them.

Milk is an important part of the High Health Diet. It provides excellent nutrition and also may lower the LDL cholesterol. Low-fat or non-fat milk or milk products are the most desirable.

Yogurt is one milk product that you should discover if you haven't already. It seems to be cut out to give you a healthful cholesterol balance. Again, favor the low-fat kind.

• Good daily amount: 1 to 1½ pints of milk or milk products.

Eggs have been controversial because of the high cholesterol content of the yolk. If you have a cholesterol problem it is certainly best to eat no more than three eggs a week, although most experts do agree that saturated fat is much more harmful than dietary cholesterol. Meanwhile, remember that you can always eat the white of an egg, which has no cholesterol at all—and which is protein of the highest quality.

I have included *alcohol in moderation* in the High Health Diet because of its HDL-raising and LDL-lowering effect. Also because many people find it pleasant and sociable. But of course you don't have to drink if you don't want to. And you should certainly not drink except moderately—say a couple of glasses of wine or the equivalent per day. I myself don't drink because I find that I can get more work done that way.

Here is a plan that spells out how the High Health Diet goes and indicates where you can look for full details.

4

The High Health Diet Plan—For Every Day

The Diet Plan outlined in this chapter represents an average of 1200 to 1300 calories per day, based on the total seven-day menu cycle, although there are variations from day to day.

MONDAY

Breakfast:

High Health Orange*
Oatmeal (or Special K) with High Health Sugar* and High Health Cream*
PLUS: piece of whole grain toast with soy margarine
Black coffee or tea with lemon

Mid Morning:

Coffee with High Health Cream*
Whole wheat or rye wafers
PLUS: soy margarine

Dip Before Lunch:

High Health Vegetables*

Lunch:

Instant Minestrone*
(You can take soup to office in a wide-mouth thermos.)
Salad of sliced tomato, basil, whole grain croutons with High Health Dressing*
(To brown-bag salad, take dressing in spill-proof container. Mix just before serving.)
Piece of whole wheat bread
Pear
Demitasse
PLUS: glass of wine

Mid Afternoon:

High Health Tea*
Whole grain toast or cracker with a little soy margarine
PLUS: 1 tablespoon honey

Dip Before Dinner:

High Health Vegetables*

Dinner:

Sole Shioyaki*
Brown rice
Endive salad with High Health Dressing*
Demitasse or Sanka
PLUS: glass of wine

Bedtime:

High Health Fruit Flip*

TUESDAY

Breakfast:

High Health Orange*

Ralston (or Total) cereal with High Health Sugar* and High Health Cream*
PLUS: piece of whole grain toast with soy margarine
Black coffee or tea with lemon

Mid Morning:
Coffee with High Health Cream*
Whole wheat or rye wafers
PLUS: soy margarine

Dip Before Lunch:
High Health Vegetables*

Lunch:
Eggsprout Soup*
Avocado and lettuce salad with High Health Dressing*
Piece of whole grain bread
Red apple
Demitasse
PLUS: glass of wine

Mid Afternoon:
High Health Tea*
Whole grain toast with a little soy margarine
PLUS: 1 tablespoon honey

Dip Before Dinner:
High Health Vegetables*

Dinner:
Shrimp Pisto*
Noodles
Escarole, chicory and radish salad with High Health Dressing*
Sangria Surprise*
Demitasse or Sanka
PLUS: glass of wine

Bedtime:
High Health Fruit Flip*

WEDNESDAY

Breakfast:

High Health Orange*
Wheatena (or Shredded Wheat) with High Health Sugar* and High Health Cream*
PLUS: piece of whole grain toast with soy margarine
Black coffee or tea with lemon

Mid Morning:

Coffee with High Health Cream*
Whole wheat or rye wafers
PLUS: soy margarine

Dip Before Lunch:

High Health Vegetables*

Lunch:

High Health Soy Soup*
Spinach and watercress salad with High Health Dressing*
Piece of whole grain bread
Small bunch of grapes
Demitasse
PLUS: glass of wine

Mid Afternoon:

High Health Tea*
Whole grain toast with a little soy margarine
PLUS: 1 tablespoon honey

Dip Before Dinner:

High Health Vegetables*

Dinner:

Baked Scallops*
Broccoli
Small boiled potato
Romaine lettuce with High Health Dressing*
Strawberry Snow*
Demitasse or Sanka

PLUS: glass of wine

Bedtime:

High Health Fruit Flip*

THURSDAY

Breakfast:

High Health Orange*

Cream of Farina (or Wheat Chex) with High Health Cream* and High Health Sugar*

PLUS: piece of whole grain toast with soy margarine

Black coffee or tea with lemon

Mid Morning:

Coffee with High Health Cream*

Whole wheat or rye wafers

PLUS: soy margarine

Dip Before Lunch:

High Health Vegetables*

Lunch:

High Health Broth*

Cole slaw

Piece of pumpernickel bread with soy margarine

Pear

Demitasse

PLUS: glass of wine

Mid Afternoon:

High Health Tea*

Whole grain toast with a little soy margarine

PLUS: 1 tablespoon honey

Dip Before Dinner:

High Health Vegetables*

Dinner:

Tuna Soufflé*

Green beans and almond slivers

Parsley carrots

Boston lettuce and watercress salad with High Health Dressing*
Peach Sherbet*
Demitasse or Sanka
PLUS: glass of wine

Bedtime:
High Health Fruit Flip*

FRIDAY

Breakfast:
High Health Orange*
Hominy grits (or Corn Flakes) with High Health Cream* and High Health Sugar*
PLUS: piece of whole grain toast with soy margarine
Black coffee or tea with lemon

Mid Morning:
Coffee with High Health Cream*
Whole wheat or rye wafers
PLUS: soy margarine

Dip Before Lunch:
High Health Vegetables*

Lunch:
Frutta Di Mare Soup*
Artichoke hearts, Italian onion and chicory salad with High Health Dressing*
Piece of whole grain bread with soy margarine
Yellow apple
Demitasse
PLUS: glass of wine

Mid Afternoon:
High Health Tea*
Whole grain toast with a little soy margarine
PLUS: 1 tablespoon honey

Dip Before Dinner:
High Health Vegetables*

Dinner:

Crab Cayenne*
Green rice
Mushrooms
Tomato, cucumber, escarole and chives salad with High Health Dressing*
Mandarin Orange in Madeira*
Demitasse or Sanka
PLUS: glass of wine

Bedtime:

High Health Fruit Flip*

SATURDAY

Breakfast:

High Health Orange*
Cream of Wheat (or Rice Chex) with High Health Sugar* and High Health Cream*
PLUS: piece of whole grain toast with soy margarine
Black coffee or tea with lemon

Mid Morning:

Coffee with High Health Cream*
Whole wheat or rye wafers
PLUS: soy margarine

Dip Before Lunch:

High Health Vegetables*

Lunch:

Winter Gazpacho*
Mimosa salad (Boston lettuce with 1 whole hard-cooked egg, grated) with High Health Dressing*
Piece of whole wheat bread
Tangelo
Demitasse
PLUS: glass of wine

Mid Afternoon:

High Health Tea*

Whole grain toast with a little soy margarine
PLUS: 1 tablespoon honey

Dip Before Dinner:
High Health Vegetables*

Dinner:
Moules Marinière*
Salad of hearts of palm, pimiento, chives, lettuce, with High Health Dressing*
Frullato*
Demitasse or Sanka
PLUS: glass of wine

Bedtime:
High Health Fruit Flip*

SUNDAY

Breakfast:
High Health Orange*
Buckwheat waffles (or pancakes) with soy margarine and a little maple sugar
Black coffee or tea with lemon

Mid Morning:
High Health Shot on the Rocks*

Lunch:
Vegetables en Brochette*
Brown rice
Grapefruit with High Health Sugar*
Demitasse
PLUS: glass of wine

Mid Afternoon:
High Health Tea*
Whole grain toast with a little soy margarine
PLUS: 1 tablespoon honey

Dip Before Dinner:
High Health Vegetables* with Caviar Dip*

Dinner:

Halibut in Herbs*
Brussels sprouts
Sautéed mushrooms
Sliced endive, watercress and escarole salad with High Health Dressing*
Pear in the Pink*
Demitasse or Sanka
PLUS: glass of wine

Bedtime:

High Health Fruit Flip*

5

High Health Food Tips: Vegetables

Vegetables play an important role in the High Health Diet, so I would like to give you a few tips about cooking them.

Boiling is the method too frequently used. If you boil vegetables, use as little water as possible and cook them for a short time. One way to cut down on the cooking time is to bring the water to boil before adding the vegetables. Keep the liquid and use it in soups.

Microwaving: Cooking vegetables in a microwave oven is rapid and conserves vitamins and minerals since very little water is used. The natural liquids found in the vegetable provide most of the necessary moisture.

Steaming is often preferable to boiling. For instance, steamed cauliflower keeps its texture much better than boiled cauliflower. And there is less nutrient loss with steaming.

Frying or *sautéing* is a good way to prepare some vegetables. Use just a little fat, moderate heat, and a good skillet.

Stir-frying is the Chinese way of sautéing. The vegetables are cut in small pieces and are done in a minute or two.

Broiling is good with a few vegetables—like eggplant brushed with some olive oil.

Baking also has its merits, especially with Idaho potatoes. If you want to save on your fuel bill, use a Dutch oven.

Braising is a method not used enough. In braising the vegetable is first browned in a small amount of fat, then liquid is added, the dish is covered. I have found that this additional liquid is superfluous. Practically all vegetables have enough water to braise well with *just* a touch of fat—and a cover.

Although canned or frozen vegetables are often economical and convenient, nothing beats the fresh product, particularly when in season. Here is a guide to vegetables around the year.

ARTICHOKES

The artichoke—the familiar globe variety—is the unopened flower bud of a member of the thistle family.

Available: Most of the year, with peak in April and May.

Look for: Plump artichokes that are very heavy for their size and have thick, fresh green scales.

Avoid: Artichokes with spreading scales (a sign of age, dryness and toughness), brown areas, grayish-black discoloration, mold on the scales, or worm damage.

Storage: Keep cold and humid and use within a few days.

ASPARAGUS

Available: March into June, and as a luxury item at other times of the year.

Look for: Stalks with the largest area of green. Fresh, firm, *closed* tips.

Avoid: Opened tips (a sign of old age) and angular or flat stalks (apt to be woody). Also steer clear of warm asparagus—it should be cold all the way to the consumer. A bunch soaking butt-end in water may be contaminated.

Storage: Keep asparagus cold and humid and use as soon as possible.

AVOCADO

Available: All year.

Look for: Avocados that are bright and fresh-looking and heavy for their size. Irregular brownish marks called scab are nothing to worry about. If the fruit is firm or hard, that is all right—it will ripen at home.

Avoid: Shriveled or bruised specimens.

Storage: Keep at room temperature until soft, then use or refrigerate.

BEANS (GREEN)

Available: All year, with peak May through August.

Look for: Fresh, bright beans as young (small) as possible.

Avoid: Flabby beans or ones with bad blemishes. Thick, fibrous pods are over-mature and tough.

Storage: Keep cold and humid and use promptly.

P.S. Yellow wax beans and large green-pole beans turn up occasionally. Try them.

BEANS, LIMA

Available: May into October, but supplies are limited.

Look for: Pods that are well filled, bright and dark green. Shelled lima beans should be plump, with a tender green or greenish-white color.

Avoid: Dried-out pods.

Storage: Keep cold and humid and use without delay. Limas are very perishable.

BEETS

Available: All year round.

Look for: Small or medium-size beets that are firm, round and a good color. If tops are fresh, use them too.

Avoid: Large beets, which are likely to be woody. Also any that are flabby, rough or shriveled.

Storage: Keep cold and humid. Use good greens (if any) immediately, and the roots within a week.

BROCCOLI

Available: All year with peak October through May. (Broccoli, a close relative of cauliflower, grows best in cool weather.)

Look for: Compact bud clusters with none opened enough to show the yellow flowers. Color can be dark green, sage green, or purple green—it all depends on the variety. Stalks should appear green and fresh.

Avoid: Broccoli with spread bud clusters, opened buds, yellowish-green color, or in a wilted condition. Thumbs down also on heads with slippery water-soaked spots on the bud cluster.

Storage: Keep cold and humid and use as soon as possible.

BRUSSELS SPROUTS

Available: Peak is September through February. The sprouts are enlarged buds that grow on a tall stem, one for each main leaf.

Look for: Fresh, bright green color, and firm compact body.

Avoid: Sprouts with yellow or yellowish-green leaves, or

leaves that are loose and wilted. Small holes may indicate worm injury.

Storage: Keep cold and humid and use promptly.

CABBAGE

Available: All year in large amounts. There are three main varieties: smooth-leaf green cabbage, crinkly-leaf green Savoy cabbage, and red cabbage. All are good for general use; the Savoy and red types are often used in cole slaws and salads. Cabbage may be sold fresh (so-called new cabbage) or from storage (the "old" cabbage).

Look for: Firm heads that are heavy for their size. The outer leaves should be green unless the head is from storage and has been trimmed.

Avoid: New cabbage with wilted or decayed outer leaves, or with leaves that are turning yellow. Worm-eaten outside leaves often mean that there is injury inside too. Storage cabbage with badly discolored, dried or decayed outer leaves is probably over-aged. Another sign of this is separation of the stems of leaves from the main stem.

Storage: Keep cold and humid and use within a week or two.

CARROTS

Available: All year round in large quantities. Most are fairly young, tender, and mild-flavored—and good to eat raw.

Look for: Firm, fresh, smooth, well-shaped carrots with a good orange color. Packs of carrots in plastic bags are usually first-rate.

Avoid: Roots with large green areas at the top or which are flabby or soft.

Storage: Keep cold and humid and use as desired.

CAULIFLOWER

Available: All year in a fairly good supply.

Look for: White or creamy white, clean, firm compact heads. A slightly granular texture doesn't affect quality as long as the flower clusters are compact. Quality has nothing to do with the size of the head. If there are any jacket leaves around the base, they should be fresh and green.

Avoid: Loose, open-flower clusters—they indicate overmaturity. Also avoid heads that are spotted or speckled or have brown areas. This can be a sign of insect injury, mold growth or decay.

Storage: Keep cold and humid. Use as soon as possible.

CELERIAC

This is often called celery root or celery knob—but it is actually just a variety of celery.

Available: All year, but mostly October through April.

Look for: Firm, clean knobs free from damage.

Storage: Keep cold and humid and use as desired.

CELERY

Most celery on the market is of the Pascal type with green outer stalks.

Available: All year in large amounts.

Look for: Fresh, crisp bunches with stalks that are thick and solid and with good heart formation. Leaves should be fresh-looking.

Avoid: Soft stems—they mean lack of freshness and often pithiness. Branches that are very hard may be stringy or woody.

A seed stem—a solid, roundish stem replacing the delicate heart branches—indicates the celery is too mature. Other things to watch out for: gray or brown on the inside surface of the larger branches where they join the base of the stalk, and "blackheart," a brown or black discoloration of the small center branches.

CHICORY, ENDIVE, ESCAROLE

Chicory (also called curly endive) has crinkly leaves with notched edges and often light yellowish leaves in the center that are milder in taste. Escarole leaves are broader and not so crinkly. Belgian endive is a creamy white, tight little plant shaped like an elongated teardrop; it is grown in the dark, so there is no green to speak of.

Available: Almost all year round, but mainly in the winter and spring.

Look for: Fresh, crisp plants with a good green color in the outer leaves (except for Belgian endive).

Avoid: Plants with brownish or yellowish discolorations.

Storage: Keep refrigerated and use within a few days.

CHINESE CABBAGE

Heads are shaped like long cylinders. Some varieties have a firm head; others are more leafy. Good for salads or cooking.

Available: All year round.

Look for: Fresh, clean, crisp plants.

Avoid: Wilted or yellowing ones.

Storage: Keep cold and humid and use within a week or so.

CHIVES

These mild relatives of the onion come in pots and provide

fresh leaves for several weeks if you take good care of them. Choose a pot that is thick and fresh-looking. Keep it in the best light available.

CORN

Sweet corn should be kept cold all the way from the field to the kettle because it turns its sugar to starch quite rapidly. This may happen to local corn which has not been cooled quickly—properly handled corn from farther away will be much fresher. Most corn now on the market is yellow.

Available: All year, but especially spring and summer.

Look for: Fresh, green husks; silk-ends free of worm injury or decay.

Avoid: Ears with underdeveloped kernels which lack color (in yellow corn); old ears with very big kernels; ears with dark yellow kernels and sunken areas; yellowed, wilted, or dried husks; stem ends that are dried-out or discolored.

Storage: Keep cool and humid. Use as soon as possible.

CUCUMBERS

Available: All year, with peak May through August.

Look for: Cucumbers of a good green color and firm the whole length. White or greenish-white areas are okay, and so are various small lumps—but the overall shape should be good. Choose medium or smaller sizes.

Avoid: Very large cucumbers—they are likely to have hard seeds. Withered or shriveled ends indicate toughness and bitter taste.

Storage: Keep cool and humid. Use within a few days.

EGGPLANT

Available: All year round, most abundant during late summer.

Look for: Uniformly dark purple eggplant, firm and heavy for its size.

Avoid: Fruit that is shriveled, soft or flabby, or with scars, cuts or worm damage. Irregular dark-brown spots indicate decay.

Storage: Keep cool and humid. Use as soon as possible.

GREENS

There are many kinds of greens. Good for cooking: kale, collards, turnip tops, beet tops, chard, mustard, broccoli leaves, Swiss chard. (For greens used mainly in salads, see Lettuce and individual entries.)

Available: One type or another all year round.

Look for: Fresh, young, tender leaves with a good green color.

Avoid: Greens with insect damage, coarse stems, seed stems, dry or yellowing leaves. Also pass by wilted or flabby leaves.

Storage: Keep cold and moist. Use as soon as possible.

HORSERADISH ROOT

Available: All year in some markets.

Look for: Firm roots with no shriveling or soft spots.

Storage: Keep cold and humid. Roots dug when the plant is still growing do not keep so well as those harvested later.

JERUSALEM ARTICHOKES

Not really an artichoke, but a relative of the sunflower. The part you eat is the tuber, which ranges up to three inches in diameter.

Available: Off and on because of irregular planting.

Look for: Good, solid tubers.

Avoid: Tubers with soft spots or excessive blemishes.

Storage: The tubers shrivel quickly when exposed to air, so keep in a plastic bag in the refrigerator. Use promptly.

KOHLRABI

A member of the cabbage family. The globe is three or four inches in diameter, with leaves like a turnip's. When young, both stem and leaves can be cooked and eaten.

Available: May through November, peaking in June and July. Supply always limited.

Look for: Firm, crisp stem, crisp and green tops.

Avoid: Wilted or shriveled specimens.

Storage: Keep cold and use within a few days.

LEEKS

A member of the onion family that used to be known as the poor-man's asparagus—by now, almost the reverse is true.

Available: All year in limited quantities, but mostly September through November and in the spring.

Look for: Green, fresh tops and medium-sized necks which are crisp and tender and well-blanched for at least two or three inches from the root.

Avoid: Yellowed, wilted tops and flabby, tough necks.

Storage: Keep cold and humid and use within a week.

LEGUMES—See Chapter 7

LETTUCE

There are many varieties to choose from, the most common being iceberg, Boston, romaine and Bibb.

Available: All year.

Look for: In iceberg and romaine, the leaves should be crisp and firm. Boston, Bibb and Simpson have softer leaves, but they should not be wilted. Leaves should have a good green color, except some of the Simpsons which tend to rusty hues.

Avoid: Leaves with ragged areas or lacking green color, a sign of over-maturity. Also heads with irregular shapes and hard bumps on top, an indication of overgrown stems.

Storage: Keep cold and humid and use within a few days.

P.S. There are quite a few different kinds of Simpson: ivy, oak, garden, bronze and others. Other salad greens besides those mentioned include rocket (the Italian rugula), dandelion, lamb's lettuce, peppergrass, sorrel. See also headings for chicory, endive, escarole; Chinese Cabbage; spinach; water-cress.

MUSHROOMS

Available: All year with peak from November to April.

Look for: Surface of the cap should be white or cream color, free of discoloration or wilting. If caps are open, the gills (rows of tissue underneath the cap) should be pink or light tan. Small to medium-sized mushrooms have a lighter flavor than the big ones.

Avoid: Dark gills indicate overripe mushrooms. Also avoid pitted or seriously discolored caps.

Storage: Keep cold and humid and use quickly.

OKRA

Available: May to October.

Look for: Bright green color, and medium size—usually two to four inches long. Pods should be young and tender and should snap easily when broken.

Avoid: Dull, dry pods as well as shriveled or discolored ones. If the tips are stiff and resist bending, this indicates toughness. Very hard pods should also be left in the bin.

Storage: Keep cool and humid and use within a few days.

ONIONS (DRY-SKINNED)

The familiar dry-skinned onions come in a number of varieties. The all-purpose yellow onion is the most common—it has a good, strong taste. The Bermuda onion is the large, flat kind with a skin that comes in various shades; it is mild and good for salads. Spanish onions are the very big ones of gray-brown color. Like the Bermudas they are mild and good raw. White onions are the junior-sized members of the family—they are milder than the yellow onions but have more bite than the Bermuda or Spanish varieties. Italian or red onions have a distinctive, pungent taste and are excellent in salads.

Garlic is also a member of the onion family, as are shallots (see Shallot entry).

Available: All year round.

Look for: Dry onions should have crisp skins that crackle. Garlic: choose a plump, solid bulb.

Avoid: Moisture at the neck-end of a dry onion indicates decay. Also avoid onions with thick, hollow woody centers, and ones that are starting to sprout. Garlic: avoid bulbs that have any soft spots or do not feel full.

Storage: Dry onions and garlic must be kept dry. They store well at room temperature.

ONIONS (GREEN)

These are ordinary onions that are harvested very young. Also known as scallions or (a little bigger) spring onions.

Available: All year, with greater abundance from May to August.

Look for: Crisp, green tops, medium-sized necks. They should be white for two or three inches up from the root.

Avoid: Wilted or discolored tops. Bruised tops should be removed, but will not affect the quality of the bulbs.

Storage: Keep cold and humid and use as soon as possible.

PARSLEY

Though generally thought of as a garnish, parsley can be used as a regular salad green. Besides the familiar crinkly kind, try the flat-leafed Italian variety—it is a little more pungent.

Available: All year.

Look for: Bright green leaves, crisp and fresh.

Avoid: Wilted or yellowed leaves.

Storage: Keep cold and humid. Don't store with stems in water. But slightly wilted leaves can be freshened if you trim off the ends first and place them in cold water for a little while

PARSNIPS

This vegetable becomes sweeter after exposure to temperatures below 40 degrees.

Available: Mainly October through April.

Look for: Small or medium-sized parsnips that are smooth and firm.

Avoid: Large, coarse, shriveled roots.

Storage: Keep cold and humid and use as desired.

PEAS, GREEN

Unfortunately, fresh green peas are rarely found on the market these days, partly because few people care to shell them, and partly because they lose their flavor and tenderness quickly if not properly stored.

Available: Formerly on the market all year, with peak from March to July.

Look for: Uniformly green pods that are well filled.

Avoid: Leathery, dried-out pods.

Storage: Should be kept cold and humid, and used as soon as possible.

PEPPERS, SWEET

Available: Throughout the year, but mostly in summer.

Look for: Firm, shiny, thick-fleshed peppers, either bright green, or with more or less red.

Avoid: Flabby peppers, or those with very thin walls, or soft watery spots on the sides.

Storage: Keep cool and humid and use within a few days.

POTATOES

Available: All year round in large quantities.

Look for: Relatively smooth and firm potatoes that have a good shape.

Avoid: Potatoes that are badly bruised or cut, or which are sprouted or shriveled. Also avoid those with a green color under the skin (it indicates sun or light burn).

Storage: Do not refrigerate, as low temperature converts the starch to sugar. Best kept in the dark at room temperature, away from heat or cold.

RADISHES

Radishes include red, white, and black varieties, either long or globular in shape. Fresh tops can be cooked and eaten.

Available: All year, with more in summer.

Look for: Smooth, firm, crisp radishes, preferably medium sized and well formed.

Avoid: Very large or flabby radishes, or those with yellow or decayed tops, which indicate over-age.

Storage: Remove tops, if any, and keep roots cold and humid.

RHUBARB

This vegetable is used as a fruit in sweetened sauces and pies. The leaves are not edible.

Available: In limited amounts through most of the year, but especially from January to June.

Look for: Firm, fresh, tender stalks with a bright appearance. Test tenderness by puncturing the stalk.

Avoid: Wilted or flabby stalks, very thick or thin stalks.

Storage: Keep refrigerated. Use promptly.

RUTABAGAS

Related to the turnip, rutabagas are slightly more elongated, have a thick neck, and are yellow in color rather than white-fleshed.

Available: All year, but mostly in winter.

Look for: Firm, heavy and generally smooth rutabagas. Size is not an indication of quality.

Avoid: Deep cuts, punctures, or any signs of decay.

Storage: Keep cold and humid and use as desired.

SHALLOTS

Shallots, onion cousins with a special taste, have a bulb made up of cloves, like garlic. Each clove is covered by a membrane.

Available: Mainly November through April.

Look for: Firm, plump, fresh-looking bulbs.

Avoid: Bulbs that are beginning to be soft and shriveled.

Storage: Refrigerate. Use when needed.

SPINACH

Available: All year, with greater abundance January through May.

Look for: Fresh, tender leaves of a good green color.

Avoid: Large leaves that are discolored, yellowish, wilted or bruised (small, yellowish-green underdeveloped heart leaves are a good sign). Avoid straggly, overgrown plants, or plants with seed stems.

Storage: Very perishable. Should be kept cold and humid, and used within a few days.

SQUASH

Summer squash refers to the varieties harvested before maturity, when the entire squash is tender and edible. Winter squash is marketed only when fully mature and has a hard shell which is not eaten.

Available: Various types are on the market all year round.

Look for: In summer squash, a glossy skin indicates tenderness. Choose well-formed, fresh-looking squash that is neither hard nor tough. Winter squash should have a hard, tough rind with no soft spots.

Avoid: A dull appearance in summer squash, as well as a hard or tough surface. In the winter varieties, avoid cuts, punctures, moldy spots or a tender rind.

Storage: Soft-skinned squash is more perishable and should be kept cold and humid, and used within a few days. The hard-shelled squashes keep longer, and may be stored at room temperature.

SWEET POTATOES

There are two types of sweet potatoes: moist and dry. The moist variety, also called yams, are the more common, and are orange-colored and quite sweet. Dry sweet potatoes are paler in color and lower in moisture.

Available: All year, but more abundant from October through April.

Look for: Smooth, well-shaped, firm tubers.

Avoid: Any signs of decay, worm holes, cuts or any defect which penetrates the skin. Even if the decayed part is cut away, the remaining portion may have a bad taste. So be especially careful in choosing sweet potatoes.

Storage: They are quite perishable, and should be kept dry and away from cold. Do not refrigerate (except after cooking).

TOMATOES

Tomatoes taste best when allowed to ripen on the vine. But if they are picked after the color has begun to change from green to pink, they are still quite flavorful. Even when picked green they will develop a red color, but without the good flavor and juiciness of tomatoes picked at a later stage.

Available: All year.

Look for: Well-formed tomatoes, which are smooth, well-ripened and reasonably unblemished.

Avoid: Bruised or overripe fruit, or fruit with green or yellow areas near the stem. Growth cracks around the stem scar should also be avoided. Surface mold, water-soaked spots and depressed areas are signs of decay.

Storage: Keep at room temperature in the open until fully ripened. Do not refrigerate until ripe.

TURNIPS

Turnips differ in color and shape, but the most popular have a purple top and white flesh. Different varieties have much the same flavor.

Available: Most of the year.

Look for: Smooth, fairly round and firm vegetables of small or medium size. Tops should be green and crisp.

Avoid: Yellowed or wilted tops which indicate old age. Very large or coarse roots. Large turnips with too many leaf scars.

Storage: Keep cold and humid and use as desired. Tops should be removed and used as soon as possible.

WATERCRESS

This small, round-leaf plant grows wild, or may be cultivated along the banks of freshwater streams and ponds. It is used as a garnish, and for salads, and has a very high vitamin A content.

Available: In limited supply through the year.

Look for: Fresh, crisp medium green leaves.

Avoid: Yellowed or wilted leaves.

Storage: Highly perishable. Keep cold and humid. Do not soak in water, but you may keep it in a plastic bag with ice. Best if used the same day as purchased.

6

High Health Food Tips: Fruits

When you think of fruit, you think of fresh fruit. Here is your fresh fruit year-round guide.

APPLES

There are a great many varieties of apples to choose from, and also many different opinions about which types should be used for what. In general, red apples are preferred for eating raw—Granny Smith apples are the one green eating apple—and green apples are used for cooking. Apples from cold storage have a better flavor than those which come right off the tree, one instance in which freshest does not necessarily mean the best.

Available: All year round in large quantities.

Look for: Firm, unbruised fruit of good color for the variety.

Avoid: Wilted or punctured fruit, or fruit that is very bruised.

Storage: Keep cold and humid and use as desired.

APRICOTS

Apricots cannot be shipped when fully ripe as they are very delicate.

Available: Mostly in June and July.

Look for: Plump, soft fruits of orange-yellow color.

Avoid: Greenish apricots, or bruised or damaged fruit.

Storage: Keep cold and humid and use within a couple of days.

BANANAS

Bananas may be eaten at various stages of ripeness—just suit your taste. Room temperature is perfect for ripening.

Available: In abundance all year round.

Look for: Plump fruit which is neither bruised nor split.

Avoid: Badly bruised, or mushy, overripe specimens.

Storage: Keep at room temperature until they are just the way you like them. You can then put them in the icebox if necessary. They will keep a couple of days under refrigeration, though the skins will turn brown.

BLACKBERRIES, RASPBERRIES, BOYSENBERRIES

Available: Mostly from June through August.

Look for: Fresh, cold, dry berries.

Avoid: Berries that are bruised or moldy and which show signs of leaking.

Storage: Keep cold and covered and use as soon as possible.

BLUEBERRIES

Available: June through August.

Look for: Plump fresh berries of good blue color. The larger sizes are best.

Avoid: Shriveled or damaged berries.

Storage: Keep cold and covered to avoid drying out. Use within two or three days.

CANTALOUPES

For cantaloupes to ripen well they must be picked at the point of maturity known as the "full slip" condition—when the stem comes off fully and smoothly. If the stem end is rough with parts of the stem still attached, the melon will probably not ripen fully, and you will taste the difference. Cantaloupes picked at full slip need three or four days at room temperature to ripen.

Available: Mostly from May through September.

Look for: A smooth stem end and firm fruit free of soft, mushy spots.

Storage: Refrigerate when ripe.

CASABA MELONS

This is a large, heavy melon, yellow when ripe, with a tough, deeply wrinkled rind. Ripeness is indicated by the yellow color and slight softening at the stem end. The flesh is soft, creamy white, and sweet and juicy.

Available: July through November in small amounts, with peak in September and October.

Storage: Keep cool and avoid drying out.

CHERRIES

Available: Late May through August.
Look for: Fresh, firm fruit that is highly colored, from bright red to black.
Avoid: Immature cherries—they will not ripen. Also sticky cherries, or cherries with any signs of decay.
Storage: Keep them cold and humid and use within two or three days.

CRANBERRIES

Available: September through December.
Look for: Firm, plump, lustrous berries, red to reddish-black.
Avoid: Dull, soft, shriveled, or sticky berries.
Storage: Refrigerate and use within a week or two. Or freeze for later use.

CRENSHAW MELONS

This is a large hybrid muskmelon which weighs 7 to 9 pounds. It has a smooth green and gold rind and bright salmon-colored meat. A ripe melon has a softened rind, particularly at the large end, and a golden color and rich aroma.
Available: From July to October, peaking in August and September.
Storage: Keep at room temperature until ripe. Then keep cool and use soon.

FIGS

Available: Mainly from August to October, in small quantities.

Look for: Soft, ripe fruit with characteristic color ranging from greenish-yellow to purple or black, depending on variety.

Avoid: Overripe figs which have a sour odor.

Storage: Keep cold and use immediately, because figs are extremely perishable.

GRAPEFRUIT

Most grapefruits are seedless nowadays—they provide much more to eat than the seedy varieties. White grapefruits tend to have a somewhat stronger flavor than the pink ones.

Available: All year.

Look for: Heavy, thin-skinned fruits that are firm and springy to the touch. Grapefruits you buy are ready to eat, as only ripe ones are shipped.

Avoid: Loose-skinned, puffy, wilted fruit. Or grapefruits which are somewhat pointed at the stem end, as these are usually thick-skinned.

Storage: Keep at room temperature or refrigerate, and use as desired.

GRAPES

Grapes are shipped only when fully matured; they do not ripen any further after they have been picked.

Look for: Smooth, plump grapes which are firmly attached to the stem. They should be well colored for the variety. White or green grapes are best when the color is slightly yellowish.

The red ones should have a good red color predominating on all or most of the berry.

Avoid: Sticky, soft or wrinkled grapes, or grapes with bleached areas at the stem end.

Storage: Keep cold and humid and use within a week.

GUAVAS

This subtropical fruit may be round, oval or pear-shaped. It has a thin green-to-yellow skin, and sometimes has a pink blush.

Available: In very scarce supply.

Storage: Keep cool and humid, and use as soon as possible.

HONEYDEW MELONS

This is a large, oval-shaped variety of the muskmelon with a very smooth rind. It ranges in color from creamy white to creamy yellow.

Available: You can find honeydews during most of the year, but the plentiful season is July through October.

Look for: A soft velvety feel, which indicates ripeness. A slight softening at the blossom end and a creamy yellow color are other signs of a fully ripened fruit.

Avoid: Melons with a hard, smooth feel, or which have a dead-white or greenish-white tinge are immature and will not sweeten. Also avoid damaged melons—check for cuts, punctures and water-soaked areas.

Storage: Keep at room temperature until fully ripe, then keep cool and humid. Best served at room temperature.

KIWI

These small, fuzzy fruits come from New Zealand. When ripe

they yield to gentle pressure.

Available: June to December.

Look for: Somewhat firm fruits, which should be allowed to ripen for a couple of days before use.

Storage: If not used immediately after ripening, refrigerate and use within a few days.

KUMQUATS

This is the smallest of the citrus fruits. It is orange-colored, and often comes with some leaves left on for looks.

Available: November through March.

Storage: Keep at room temperature or refrigerate.

LEMONS

Available: All year in abundance.

Look for: Firm fruit, heavy for its size, with a fine-textured skin and rich yellow color.

Avoid: Fruit that is beginning to look old.

Storage: Lemons keep better at room temperature than refrigerated if used within a week or so.

LIMES

Available: All year.

Look for: Firm fruit with good green color.

Avoid: Limes that have started to shrivel.

Storage: Same as lemons, but do not last as well.

MANGOES

This tropical fruit is round to oval, and weighs half a pound to a pound. Its smooth skin is green with yellow and red areas which spread as the fruit ripens.

Available: May through August.

Avoid: Wilted mangoes, or mangoes that have any pitting, black spots, or grayish discoloration.

Storage: Keep at room temperature until very soft, then refrigerate.

NECTARINES

Peach-like inside, plum-like outside. Like peaches, nectarines must be picked when ripe, or almost ripe.

Available: Mostly June through September.

Look for: Highly colored fruit that is smooth, plump and unblemished, with a slight softening along the seam. Firm to moderately hard fruits usually ripen in a few days at room temperature.

Avoid: Fruit that is soft, overripe, or shows any sign of decay. Hard, dull nectarines are immature and will not ripen properly.

Storage: Ripen at room temperature, then keep cold and humid.

ORANGES

Oranges are ripe before they are picked (it's the law). Color does not mean anything, as fully matured oranges often turn green late in the marketing season. Florida oranges may be colored artificially with a harmless dye—they are then stamped "color added." Russeting—a tan, brown, or blackish mottling of the skin—does not affect quality, and in fact often occurs on oranges of excellent taste.

Available: All year. December to May is the most abundant season for both Florida (juice oranges) and California (navel especially). Valencias are good to eat in the summer when navels may be scarce.

Look for: Firm, heavy oranges with fresh, bright-looking skin. Navels have a coarser skin than the fine-skinned Florida oranges.

Avoid: Light, puffy, or spongy oranges, as they lack juice. Dull, dry skin indicates inferior taste. A hard peel is likely to be thick.

Storage: Keep at room temperature or refrigerate. Use as desired.

PAPAYAS

Available: All year in small amounts, peaking in May and June.

Look for: Papayas of moderate size—they usually have more flavor than very large ones. Fruit should be somewhat pear-shaped. The skin should be smooth and unbroken, with no large green areas.

Avoid: Fruits showing any signs of deterioration or shriveling.

Storage: Keep at room temperature until ripe, then refrigerate and use as soon as possible.

PEACHES

Peaches do not ripen very much after picking. So buy them as near tree-ripe as possible. Green fruits do not ripen properly and have a poor taste.

Available: June through September.

Look for: Fairly firm peaches, with a yellow or at least cream-colored ground color.

Avoid: Very firm or hard peaches with a green color. Also very soft, overripe peaches, or any with large bruises or any sign of decay.

Storage: Hold at room temperature until soft, then refrigerate and use as soon as possible.

PEARS

It is difficult to tell when pears are ripe—they ripen from the inside out, and by the time they are soft outside, the inside is probably mushy and tasteless. Pears are picked mature but hard, and are best when ripened off the tree, at room temperature.

Available: Different varieties are in season at different times of year.

Look for: Firm pears of all varieties. Choose pears which have begun to soften *slightly* around the stem to be sure they will ripen well.

Avoid: Pears that are misshapen, shriveled, soft or that have a dull skin.

Storage: Ripen at room temperature, then keep cold and humid and eat as soon as possible.

PERSIAN MELONS

Similar to cantaloupes, but rounder, and about the same size as honeydews. The flesh is thick and orange.

Available: August and September.

Look for: A smooth stem end ("full slip") and a yellowish ground color. When ripe, the rind gives under slight pressure.

Avoid: Overripeness, indicated by a deep yellow rind color, softening over the entire rind, and large bruised areas. A rough stem end indicates the fruit was picked too soon and will not ripen properly. Mold, particularly in the stem scar, is a sign of decay.

Storage: After softening at room temperature, keep cold and humid and eat as soon as possible.

PINEAPPLES

Pineapples must be picked when hard, but are usually ripe by the time you find them in the store.

Available: All year round, but especially from March through June.

Look for: Fruit that is heavy for its size, and as large as possible. The crown leaves should look fresh and be a deep green color. Fragrance is a good sign, so is a very slight separation of the eyes. Plump, glossy eyes, firmness and a bright color are also indications of maturity.

Avoid: Fruit with brown leaves, discolored or soft spots. Signs of decay include traces of mold, an unpleasant odor, and eyes that are watery and dark in color.

Storage: Keep cold and humid and use quickly.

PLANTAINS

Often described as a large, starchy type of banana which does not become sweet, although, in fact, there are plantains which do sweeten. It is usually the cooking type that is available in this country.

Available: All year in small amounts.

Look for: Fruit that looks like unripe bananas.

Storage: Keep at room temperature.

PLUMS AND PRUNES

Available: Mainly from June until September.

Look for: Good color for the variety, and a fairly firm to slightly soft stage of ripeness.

Avoid: Immature fruit which is relatively hard and poorly

colored. Shriveled, punctured or discolored specimens. Any that are excessively soft, leaking or decaying.

Storage: Allow to ripen fully at room temperature, then keep cold and humid and use as soon as possible.

POMEGRANATES

Available: From late September into November, with greatest abundance in October.

Look for: Fruit with pink or bright red rind.

Avoid: Pomegranates that look hard and dry.

Storage: Keep cold and humid.

PUMPKINS

Available: Mostly in late October.

Look for: A good orange-golden color, a hard rind, and fruit that is heavy for its size.

Avoid: Fruit with cuts or severe bruises.

Storage: Keep cool until use.

STRAWBERRIES

Available: All year, but in best supply from April through June.

Look for: Fresh, clean berries with a bright solid red color. The cap stem should be still attached. The medium sizes are usually the most flavorful.

Avoid: Small misshapen berries, or extremely large ones. Berries with large uncolored or seedy areas, a dull shrunken appearance or soft, mushy texture. Stained containers indicate leakage and decay.

Storage: Strawberries are highly perishable. Keep them cold and humid and use as soon as possible.

TANGELOS

This fruit is a cross between mandarin orange and grapefruit.

Available: Late October through January.

Look for: Firm fruit, heavy for size, with a light orange color and thin skin.

Avoid: Badly blemished, lightweight tangelos.

Storage: May be kept at room temperature, or cold and humid, depending on length of storage.

TANGERINES

Available: From late November until early March, peaking in December and January.

Look for: Tangerines that are heavy for their size and have a deep orange or almost red color. A loose, puffy skin is normal.

Avoid: Soft or water-soaked areas or mold mean decay. Also avoid very pale yellow or greenish fruit which is likely to lack flavor.

Storage: Highly perishable. Keep cold and humid and use as soon as possible.

WATERMELONS

Available: Mostly May into September.

Look for: In cut pieces, firm juicy flesh, a good red color, and dark brown or black seeds. Uncut: The rind should be neither shiny nor dull, the ends of the fruit should be rounded, and the underside should have a creamy color.

Avoid: Immature fruit, indicated by green or white underside, or extremely hard rind, as a watermelon does not ripen after it comes off the vine. Also avoid pieces with pale flesh, white streaks, and whitish seeds. Dry, mealy or stringy, watery flesh are signs of age.

Storage: Uncut melons may be kept at room temperature. Cut chunks should be refrigerated.

For all fruits and vegetables, keep an eye out for what is in season. This chart will help you. It shows the monthly availability of 65 different fruits and vegetables. Each figure represents a percentage of the total annual supply. For instance, artichokes rate 22 in April—meaning that 22 percent of the annual artichoke crop is on the market then: a big artichoke month. An average month would be 8 or 9. Higher than that means above-average supplies. Less means below average.

MONTHLY AVAILABILITY EXPRESSED AS PERCENTAGE OF TOTAL ANNUAL SUPPLY

COMMODITY	Jan. %	Feb. %	Mar. %	Apr. %	May %	June %	July %	Aug. %	Sept. %	Oct. %	Nov. %	Dec. %
APPLES, all	9	9	10	9	8	6	3	4	9	12	10	11
Washington	10	10	11	10	10	7	5	3	5	8	10	11
New York	9	9	11	10	9	5	2	3	9	11	11	9
Michigan	13	12	13	11	7	2	*	2	6	11	11	11
California	5	5	7	6	3	*	3	15	26	16	8	5
Virginia	11	10	10	5	2	1	1	2	14	17	14	13
APRICOTS					7	58	29	6				
ARTICHOKES	3	5	11	22	21	10	4	4	4	6	5	5
ASPARAGUS	*	7	25	34	20	9	*	*	1	2	1	
AVOCADOS, all	9	7	9	8	8	8	8	8	8	8	10	9
California	8	8	10	10	10	10	9	8	7	6	6	8
BANANAS	8	7	9	9	9	8	8	8	8	8	9	9
BEANS, SNAP, all	6	5	6	9	10	12	11	10	9	8	7	7
Florida	11	9	14	20	14	2	*		*	2	13	14
BEETS	5	5	8	7	7	11	13	12	10	9	7	6
BERRIES, MISC.**					1	20	38	16	12	9	4	
BLUEBERRIES					2	24	48	24	2			
BROCCOLI	9	8	12	8	8	8	7	5	7	8	9	11
BRUSSELS SPROUTS	13	12	11	8	4	*	*	2	6	14	16	13
CABBAGE, all	9	8	10	9	9	9	7	7	8	8	8	8
Florida	16	14	23	20	15	3	*			*	1	7
Texas	16	14	15	13	10	4	2	1	1	2	8	14
California	10	9	11	9	11	11	7	6	5	7	7	7
New York	10	7	5	2	1	1	8	10	12	15	17	12
North Carolina	1			*	12	31	8	8	8	7	15	10
CANTALOUPES, all	*	*	3	4	9	19	24	23	12	4	1	*
California					*	14	28	32	17	6	2	*
Mexico	*	2	16	28	44	9	*			*	*	*
Texas					18	47	21	11	2	*	*	
CARROTS, all	10	9	10	9	8	8	7	7	8	8	8	8
California	10	8	9	9	10	11	9	7	6	6	7	10
Texas	14	15	21	16	8	2	1	1	2	3	7	10

COMMODITY	Jan.	Feb.	Mar.	Apr.	May	June	July	Aug.	Sept.	Oct.	Nov.	Dec.
	%	%	%	%	%	%	%	%	%	%	%	%
CAULIFLOWER, all	8	7	9	9	8	7	6	6	8	12	11	9
California	9	7	10	11	10	8	6	6	6	7	10	10
CELERY, all	9	8	9	9	8	8	7	7	7	7	11	10
California	7	7	8	7	7	9	8	8	7	8	13	11
Florida	17	14	18	18	15	7	1			*	2	7
Michigan						*	18	29	32	18	2	*
CHERRIES, SWEET					6	42	46	6				
CHINESE CABBAGE	9	9	8	9	8	8	8	8	8	8	8	9
COCONUTS	10	8	8	8	6	5	5	7	8	9	12	14
CORN, SWEET, all	3	2	4	7	16	18	17	14	7	5	4	3
Florida	5	4	5	13	26	23	5	*	*	5	7	6
California					9	30	23	18	10	6	4	*
New York							8	48	37	7		
CRANBERRIES	*								10	25	45	20
CUCUMBERS, all	6	5	6	9	11	13	12	9	7	8	8	6
Florida	4	1	3	18	26	11	1		*	8	17	10
Mexico	23	22	22	12	3	*	*			*	2	15
California	*	*	1	3	11	17	20	16	13	10	6	2
EGGPLANT	9	7	8	10	8	8	8	9	8	8	9	8
ESCAROLE-ENDIVE	9	8	11	10	9	8	7	7	7	7	8	9
GARLIC	8	8	9	9	7	9	10	9	9	8	7	7
GRAPEFRUIT, all	12	12	13	11	9	6	3	3	4	7	10	10
Florida	12	12	13	13	10	5	2	*	2	10	11	10
Texas	19	19	17	11	5	*			*	4	10	14
Western	4	5	5	7	12	16	17	18	10	2	3	3
GRAPES, table	3	2	4	3	2	6	10	19	19	15	10	7
GREENS***	10	10	11	10	9	7	5	5	7	8	9	9
HONEYDEWS	1	1	2	3	6	15	12	19	21	14	4	2
LEMONS	8	7	8	8	9	10	10	10	8	7	7	8
LETTUCE, all	7	8	9	9	9	9	9	9	8	8	8	7
California	8	8	8	7	10	10	9	9	9	8	7	7
Arizona	11	7	11	23	7	1	*	*	*	3	15	21
Florida	16	13	21	21	9	1				*	6	12
Ohio	6	6	9	7	6	8	12	12	9	9	9	7
LIMES	7	4	6	6	8	11	12	12	10	7	8	9
MANGOES	*	2	4	6	14	24	24	19	5	1		
MUSHROOMS	9	8	9	8	9	8	7	8	8	8	9	9
NECTARINES	*	1	*		*	19	32	30	16	1		
OKRA	2	3	8	8	10	14	15	15	11	8	4	2
ONIONS, DRY, all	8	7	8	8	9	9	8	9	9	9	8	8
Texas	*	*	5	24	27	14	13	11	3	1	*	*
Idaho-Oregon	17	13	12	2	*			2	11	15	14	13
California	3	1	1	1	11	20	20	17	9	7	5	5
New York	12	9	11	6	2	*	1	7	15	12	12	12
ONIONS, GREEN	7	7	9	10	11	9	9	8	7	7	8	8
ORANGES, all	12	11	12	11	10	7	5	4	4	5	8	11
Western	9	10	12	12	11	8	6	5	6	5	6	10
Florida	17	13	12	10	9	6	3	1	1	4	10	14

COMMODITY	Jan. %	Feb. %	Mar. %	Apr. %	May %	June %	July %	Aug. %	Sept. %	Oct. %	Nov. %	Dec. %
PAPAYAS, HAWAII	7	7	7	6	8	10	9	8	9	10	10	9
PARSLEY & HERBS****	8	7	10	8	7	7	7	8	8	8	11	11
PARSNIPS	12	11	12	9	7	5	4	3	7	11	10	9
PEACHES, all	*	*	*	*	6	23	29	27	13	1		
California					5	23	29	26	15	2		
South Carolina					2	30	49	18	1			
Georgia					19	50	28	3	*			
New Jersey						*	14	54	31	*		
PEARS, all	7	6	7	6	5	4	4	13	16	14	10	8
California	1	*	*	*			11	34	27	19	6	1
Washington	8	8	9	8	6	3	1	6	15	14	12	10
Oregon	14	14	12	7	4	1		*	3	15	16	13
PEAS, GREEN	12	12	13	13	12	12	10	6	5	2	1	2
PEPPERS, all	8	7	8	7	8	10	11	9	9	8	8	7
Florida	15	9	10	14	16	14	1			*	6	15
California				*	2	7	13	15	20	28	14	1
Mexico	19	24	25	13	5	2	1	1	1	1	2	6
PERSIMMONS										33	48	19
PINEAPPLES	7	7	11	10	12	12	9	7	6	5	7	7
PLANTAINS	7	7	6	8	8	9	9	11	10	9	6	10
PLUMS-PRUNES	*	*	*		1	15	33	32	15	2		
POMEGRANATES								2	9	72	15	2
POTATOES, all	9	8	9	8	9	8	8	8	8	9	8	8
California	5	5	5	4	9	23	23	9	5	4	4	4
Idaho	13	12	13	13	13	7	1	*	1	6	10	10
Maine	13	12	15	17	15	5	*	*	1	3	8	10
Colorado	12	10	12	11	7	*	*	6	9	11	10	11
North Dakota	15	13	14	12	5	1	*	*	2	9	14	14
PUMPKINS	1	1	2	2	2	2	*	*	3	83	2	1
RADISHES	8	8	10	11	11	8	8	7	6	6	9	8
RHUBARB	8	15	16	23	21	9	3	1	1	1	1	1
SPINACH, all	9	9	11	9	9	8	7	6	7	8	8	9
California	9	10	12	10	9	7	7	7	6	7	8	8
SQUASH, all	8	6	6	7	8	9	10	9	9	11	10	7
California	4	3	3	8	10	12	11	10	10	13	11	5
Florida	11	9	11	15	15	3	*	1	1	6	14	14
STRAWBERRIES, all	3	5	8	18	29	16	7	5	4	2	1	2
California		*	3	22	35	18	9	6	4	2	*	*
Mexico	21	25	29	5						*	5	14
SWEET POTATOES, all	9	8	8	7	5	3	3	5	9	11	19	13
North Carolina	9	8	10	10	7	4	1	1	6	12	19	13
Louisiana	9	8	9	6	2	*	5	11	11	11	16	12
California	8	7	8	8	5	4	3	3	7	10	20	17
TANGELOS	23	4	*							*	33	39
TANGERINES	21	8	7	4	2	*			*	5	20	32

COMMODITY	Jan.	Feb.	Mar.	Apr.	May	June	July	Aug.	Sept.	Oct.	Nov.	Dec.
	%	%	%	%	%	%	%	%	%	%	%	%
TOMATOES, all	7	6	8	8	11	11	11	9	7	8	7	7
California	1	*		*	1	8	17	16	16	22	13	5
Mexico	13	17	22	20	16	5	*	*	*	*	2	3
Florida	14	8	10	12	20	13	*	*		*	6	17
Ohio			1	6	18	20	24	11	5	6	7	2
TURNIPS & RUTABAGAS	12	10	10	8	6	4	4	6	7	11	13	9
Canada	11	10	9	7	3	1	1	4	10	12	19	13
WATERMELONS	*	*	1	3	10	28	31	20	5	1	*	*

*Supply is less than 0.5% of annual total.

**Mostly raspberries, blackberries and dewberries.

***Includes kale, kohlrabi, collards, cabbage sprouts, dandelion, mustard and turnip tops, poke salad, bok choy and rappini.

****Includes also parsley root, anise, basil, chives, dill, horseradish and others.

7

High Health Food Tips: Beans, Grains, Nuts

Legumes, the family of beans and peas, are good for your health, and are also an excellent food bargain when you buy them in their traditional dry form. They are a rich source of protein, especially when combined with rice or other grains (thus forming "complete" proteins, those containing all eight essential amino acids). Legumes also have good amounts of thiamine and riboflavin and many contain a healthy amount of calcium. Legumes are rich in iron—a cup of cooked dried peas or beans supplies about a fourth of the iron needed daily by a woman, and a third of that required by a man.

BUYING LEGUMES

Most legumes are officially inspected at some point before marketing, although retail packages unfortunately do not always carry the Federal or State grade. Beans, peas and lentils are graded according to shape, size, color, damage and foreign matter. The greater the uniformity of color and size, the higher the Federal grade will be. Larger quantities of foreign matter, off-color and uneven size mean lower Federal grades. Some legumes are graded by State agencies, which use guidelines similar to the Federal ones.

You can check these qualities yourself if you do not find packages marked with Federal or State grades. Just choose legumes that are packaged in cellophane or have a see-through window, and check for color, size and visible defects. Beans, peas and lentils should have a bright, uniform color. Loss of color does not affect the actual eating quality, but it does indicate long storage and lack of freshness. Uniformity of size is important as larger beans cook more slowly than smaller ones. In general, avoid legumes with cracked seed coats, a good deal of foreign matter and pinholes (they are caused by insects).

STORING

Dried peas, beans and lentils will keep for several months if stored in a dry, cool (50 to 70 degrees F) place. Remember that older legumes take longer to cook, so do not mix the contents of packages bought at different times. Once the package is opened, store any unused portion in a glass or metal container with a close-fitting cover.

COOKING

Beans, peas and lentils should be washed before use. Pick them over to remove any small stones or other foreign matter.

Soak dry beans and whole peas first to reduce cooking time. Do not soak lentils or split peas used in soup, although you may soak split peas used for other purposes. To soak beans and whole peas, first boil them in water for two minutes, remove from heat, then soak one hour and they are ready for cooking.

If you wish to soak beans or peas overnight, it is still a good idea to boil them first for two minutes, as this eliminates hard skins, and will also keep them from souring.

Do not add salt until after soaking as this toughens the skin and increases cooking time.

To avoid breaking the skins, boil gently and stir very little. Pressure-cooking is all right for some dry beans and peas, but do not use this method for those which normally cook in a short time, such as lentils, split peas and black-eyed peas. Do not forget that dried legumes expand while cooking—a cup of the dried product will yield 2 to 2¾ cups of cooked beans, depending on the kind.

Below is a list of the main types of legumes, with tips on using them.

Black beans Also called black-turtle-soup beans, these are used to make salads and soups. Often used in Oriental and Mediterranean dishes.

Great Northern beans Used in soups, salads, casseroles.

Chick-peas Also called garbanzo beans, they have a nutty flavor, and can be pickled in vinegar and oil for salads. Also excellent as a main dish served with rice or some other grain. Hummos, a delicious Middle Eastern dish, is a creamy dip made of cooked, mashed chick-peas mixed with sesame paste (ground sesame seeds, called tahini, a product you can buy in specialty stores).

Black-eyed peas Small, oval-shaped, cream-colored beans with a black spot on the side. Good as a main dish.

Lima beans Good as a main dish vegetable or in casseroles. They are broad and flat and come in various sizes.

Kidney beans These are red, kidney-shaped and quite large. They are used to make spicy bean salads and various Mexican dishes.

Navy beans This is a broad term which covers various types of beans, including pea beans, Great Northern, and small white beans.

Pinto beans Like Great Northern beans, but smaller. Excellent for soups. They do not lose their shape even when cooked tender.

Red and pink beans The red beans have a stronger flavor than the pink ones. Both are used for Mexican dishes.

Peas Green and yellow whole peas and split peas vary a little in taste, but are used interchangeably in many recipes. All make delicious soups (remember that split peas should not be soaked when used for this purpose). The various types of dry peas can be served in many ways: they are delicious when simply boiled and served with a little margarine, but can also be used for more elaborate preparations, including dips, patties, croquettes, purees and soufflés.

Dry split peas These have had the skins removed, and then are broken in half by a special machine. They are used mainly for split pea soup, but they also combine well with many different foods.

Dry whole peas Used for soups, casseroles, puddings, dips, hors d'oeuvres and vegetable side dishes.

Yellow dry peas Have a milder flavor than other types of peas, and are most popular in the eastern and southern parts of the country.

Green dry peas Have a more distinctive flavor than the yellow varieties.

Lentils These small, disc-shaped legumes have been known for thousands of years. They are easy to prepare—they only take about thirty minutes. If you wish to drain the cooked lentils, do not discard the liquid—it is rich in vitamins and minerals and can be used in soup. Lentils are delicious in salads and soups, and make a hearty main dish, cooked with onions and spices and served with rice.

Cooking lentils is easy. Soak in cold water to cover 1 to 2 hours prior to cooking. Drain. Put 2 cups of lentils in a heavy saucepan, add 5 cups of water and just a pinch of salt. Bring to a boil, cover tightly and reduce heat. Simmer gently for about a half hour, then drain off liquid. You may add a little olive oil, or vary the flavor with a bay leaf, garlic, onion or other vegetables during cooking.

THE GREAT SOYBEAN

Soybeans are a terrific food—and very big business. Soy originated in China, but today it is the leading cash crop in this country.

Soybeans come in many forms, all of which can make a valuable addition to your diet. They are rich in protein, and the quality of the protein is excellent since it contains all the essential amino acids. Fresh green soybeans are a good source of vitamins and minerals, including vitamin A, thiamine, riboflavin, calcium, phosphorus and iron. The oil in soybeans is high in polyunsaturated fat, and, as I mentioned earlier, soy seems to have an especially good effect on your cholesterol balance.

Fresh soybeans are available in some parts of the country in late summer and fall, but the dried variety is found all year round. The kind used for cooking is milder in flavor, and somewhat larger, than the so-called field-type soybean, which goes for oil and flour production.

Fresh soybeans They are ready to use when the pods are bright green. To shell, first cover the pods with boiling water and let stand five minutes. Then drain and cool. Break the pods crosswise and squeeze out the beans. You should get almost 2 cups of shelled beans from a pound in the pod. Fresh soybeans should be used as soon as possible as they do not keep very long. If you must store them a while, put them in a covered container and place in your refrigerator. For extended storage you can blanch and then freeze them.

Green soybeans are also available in cans. They are already cooked, and you just heat and season them as you wish.

Dry soybeans You prepare these the same way as other dried beans. First sort them and remove cracked, shriveled or discolored beans. To soak, use 4 cups of water for 1 cup of dry beans, boil a couple of minutes, then remove from the heat and let soak for about an hour. Then add a pinch of salt, cover and simmer gently for about two to three hours or until tender. If you want you can add just a little oil to the water to reduce foaming.

Dry soybeans should be stored in a cool, dry place. When cooked, they will keep about a week in the refrigerator.

Soybean sprouts You can buy these sprouted or sprout them yourself at home from any dry soybeans. Before using, rinse and drain well. Remove any beans that are discolored. The sprouts can be stored in the refrigerator for three to five days in a closed plastic bag. Soybean sprouts can be eaten raw in a salad. Or you can parboil them for just a few minutes and then add to other hot dishes. The sprouts are a good source of vitamin C, so cook as little as possible—some vitamin C is lost when exposed to heat.

Soy flour This is a very useful addition to baked products as it greatly increases their nutritive value. It also gives them a better texture, a richer color, and keeps them tender and moist. Soy flour cannot entirely take the place of all-purpose flour because it does not have any gluten, the substance that holds baked products together. Soy flour must be mixed with other flours.

There are three kinds of flour made from soybeans.

The full-fat flour has all the fat which is found in the whole bean. It is over 35 percent protein and about 20 percent fat.

Low-fat flour is about 6 percent fat and about 45 percent protein.

Defatted flour has less than 1 percent fat and is about 50 percent protein.

Full-fat flour has been the type you generally find in stores, but there is such a growing interest in soy that the other varieties will soon become widely available. One caution—be sure to store soy flour of the full-fat type in a cool, dry place. If the temperature is too high, it may become rancid.

Soybean curd Also called tofu, this product has been used in Oriental cooking for thousands of years. Fresh bean curd is available in many grocery stores usually in the fresh produce area and specialty markets—in square cakes which are kept in water. Buy curd which is firm and unbroken. You can store it for several days. Just cover with water and put it in the refrigerator, preferably in a tightly covered receptacle. Change the water daily and rinse before using. Tofu is very bland and can be added to practically any dish—hot or cold, salads, main dishes. It takes seasoning very well. You can also make tofu puddings and tofu pies.

In case there is no store with fresh tofu in your neighborhood, see if you can get hold of packaged instant bean curd powder. If you are very ambitious, you can get a kit to manufacture tofu from the bean.

Soy milk You can get soy milk in dry, concentrated forms that are ready to use. Soy milk can be used in place of cow's milk in many recipes—some people like to use half soy and half regular skim milk. You can also prepare soy milk at home from the bean, but it is a good deal of work. Soy milk has about the same protein content as cow's milk, but contains less calcium, phosphorus and vitamin A. The fat content is a good deal less—it is about a half to two-thirds of that of whole milk. Commercial soy milk is often fortified with vitamins and minerals to more closely approximate cow's milk.

Soybean oil When processed, soybean oil is light in color and mild in flavor and can be used in any recipe. Unrefined soybean oil has a strong flavor and is dark brown—it may alter the flavor and color of the product. Many commercial oils contain soybean oil, as do many margarines. Soybean oil is best kept in the refrigerator after you have opened it.

GRAINS

Grains—or cereals—are the world's most important food. Here is a quick checklist of some kinds that are available.

Wheat This comes in a number of exotic varieties which include bulgur, the Middle Eastern delicacy, of which the United States is now the main producer. Bulgur is cracked wheat from which some of the bran has been removed. You can have it hot, like a nutty version of rice, or cold, as in the wonderful Lebanese tabbouli salad.

Another wheat variant is the North African couscous, which is actually what we call semolina. It is made from durum wheat which is ground into granules.

Wheat germ is the delicate embryo of the seed and can be

used with practically any salad or main dish.

Oats Dr. Samuel Johnson used to make fun of James Boswell because of the Scottish habit of eating oats, which Johnson considered fit only for horses. But the good doctor was greatly mistaken, as oats are one of the most nutritious grains. Rolled oatmeal is the form that is most readily available today.

Buckwheat This has nothing to do with wheat. It's a different grain that is used widely in Russia, especially in a dish called kasha.

Corn Corn is America's contribution to the grain kingdom. There are many varieties of cornmeal available. Corn makes a very pleasing dish, but its nutritional content is not up to most other grains. Enrichment makes up for some of its deficiencies.

Barley This is a grain that deserves to be used much more than it is. You can get barley grain in three sizes. It is particularly good in soups.

Millet Another grain that deserves wider use. It comes from Asia and can be cooked like any other whole cereal.

Rye Most of this grain goes into whiskey or flour, but you can find rye groats (coarsely ground grain) which you can cook like buckwheat.

Rice There are innumerable varieties of this grain, which is the great staple of the Far East. The two main groups are long grain and short grain. With the long-grain varieties the grains remain separated much better. Short-grain rice is likely to get soft and coagulate. Brown rice is rice from which only the inedible husks have been removed. It has more nourishment than polished rice, it is cheaper, and it has more taste. It is of interest that several serious deficiency diseases have plagued Far Eastern countries where people insisted on white rice as a status symbol.

Wild rice An absolutely delicious grain that isn't a rice at all. It comes from grass that grows in northern marshes in the United States. By law the Indians are the only persons allowed to gather it. In recent years the price of wild rice has soared, but it is still worth the price—if only for special occasions.

Cooking Cereals are all cooked much the same way. The

only thing that really varies is the amount of liquid you add. This depends mainly on how fine the grains are after processing. Whole grain takes longer than cracked grain, and cracked grain takes longer than ground. The package directions are the best to follow. Some people like cooking over direct heat after the water has first been brought to a boil. Others prefer the longer method—start over direct heat, but then shift to a double boiler. The first method may take fifteen minutes or so, the second, twenty-five or thirty minutes.

Flours The all-purpose white flour is a very good staple, and enrichment has restored some of the key nutrients lost in refining. Be sure to explore the many other kinds of flour—whole wheat flour, cracked wheat flour, wheat germ flour, gluten flour, and flours made from grains other than wheat—rye, buckwheat, oats, rice, barley. Also try some of the flours made from non-cereals, like cottonseed flour, lima bean flour, potato flour, peanut flour, carob flour. They are particularly good mixed with other flavors.

Breads Try making your own. And try all the wonderful traditional varieties brought over from Europe and still made in so many American neighborhoods.

NUTS

Using nuts can make a special contribution to a healthful diet. They are rich in flavor, crunchy in texture—and nutritious as well. Most nuts on the market have about 10 to 25 protein. Peanuts are the highest in protein with 25 percent. (Peanuts, incidentally, are not really nuts. They are a legume, a member of the bean family.)

One thing to remember is that nuts are a very concentrated form of calories because of their relatively high fat content. Calories per ounce for shelled nuts go from 165 for peanuts to 195 for pecans (except for chestnuts, which are a relatively low 55 calories). However, the fat in nuts has a healthful balance, with the polyunsaturates outweighing the saturates in all cases. This is specially true of walnuts, which have a polyunsaturated to saturated ratio of 8 or 9 to 1. Many nuts, such as peanuts, have monounsaturate fat as their main oil, so that they are similar to olive oil in their fat balance.

If you look at the following chart, you will see what I mean. The walnuts have lots of linoleic acid, the polyunsaturated oil that is so prevalent in the vegetable kingdom. But starting with filberts as you go down the list, you will notice that oleic acid—the most frequent monounsaturate in vegetable foods—is the predominant fat in the nut. You will also see that there is always a good balance of polyunsaturate over saturate—except for the cashew. But the quantities then are so low that this does not matter much.

Type Nut	Amount (gms.)	Total Fat (gms.)	Total Saturated Fatty Acids (gms.)	Unsaturated Fatty Acids: Oleic (monounsaturated) (gms.)	Unsaturated Fatty Acids: Linoleic (polyunsaturated) (gms.)
English walnut	28 (1 oz.)	18.1	1.3	2.7	11.2
Black walnut	"	16.8	1.0	5.9	8.1
Filberts	"	17.7	.9	9.6	2.8
Almonds	"	15.4	1.2	10.3	3.1
Pecans	"	20.2	1.4	12.7	4.0
Pistachio	"	15.2	1.5	10.0	2.9
Peanuts	"	14.1	3.1	6.1	4.1
Peanut butter	"	14.2	2.6	6.7	4.0
Brazil	"	19.0	3.8	9.1	4.9
Cashew	"	13.0	2.2	9.1	.9

United States Department of Agriculture Publications

Buying nuts You can buy nuts shelled or unshelled with the exception of cashews, which are always sold shelled. Most nuts are not roasted if they are sold in the shell. Shelled nuts on the other hand come raw, roasted or blanched. Roasted nuts may be salted or unsalted. Shelled nuts also come in different shapes—whole kernels, broken pieces, slivers, or ground.

There is a great variety in prices, so be sure to shop around. The shelled varieties obviously cost more, but they are convenient. Slivered nuts save time if you are going to use them as a garnish, as for instance with *sole amandine*.

If you're getting nuts in the shell, be sure to avoid moldy specimens as they may not be safe. Shelled nuts should be plump and reasonably uniform in size and color. Limp or shriveled nuts are likely to be stale. You can check on this easily as shelled nuts are usually sold in transparent packages.

Storage Most nuts must be shielded from the air's oxygen and also from high temperatures lest they become rancid. Nuts in the shell quite naturally keep their quality better than shelled nuts. Unroasted nuts keep better than roasted ones.

Nuts in the shell are fine in a bowl at room temperature for a short time. For longer storage they should be in a cool, dry place. Shelled nuts are best kept in well-closed containers in the refrigerator. There they will stay fresh for several months.

Shelled nuts in a can that has not been opened keep well in a cool place but last even better if you put them in the refrigerator. You can also freeze nuts—shelled or unshelled—in freezer containers at 0 degrees F or below.

Chestnuts are quite perishable at room temperature. But they can be stored for several months in the refrigerator in a loosely covered container.

Preparation If you have trouble cracking nuts which have a hard shell, try soaking them first in warm water for several hours. Then apply nutcracker, hammer, or whatever other blunt instrument you favor.

If the nutmeat has a thick skin, you may want to remove it to improve flavor and appearance. You can do this by dipping the shelled nuts in boiling water briefly—the process known as blanching—or by roasting. Allow about three minutes for almonds or peanuts if you are blanching them. Chestnuts also take about two or three minutes for blanching.

Roasting or toasting nuts can enhance the flavor as well as help you get rid of the skins. Five to ten minutes in a moderate oven (350 degrees F) or until lightly browned is enough. You can also toast the nuts in a heavy pan. Allow ten to fifteen minutes or until lightly browned. Stir frequently. Nuts should be cooled on a paper towel.

To roast peanuts in the shell, allow fifteen to twenty minutes in a moderate oven. Chestnuts should first be slashed with a sharp knife on the flat side and then placed with the cut up on a baking sheet. Roast in a hot oven (400 degrees F) until they are tender, about twenty minutes.

Nuts can be used in all sorts of dishes—salads, soups, main dishes, desserts. They are also delicious in breads.

8

High Health Food Tips: Milk

Milk and milk products are a key part of the High Health Diet. Here is a quick rundown (cheeses later):

Whole milk: Grade A whole milk contains at least 3.25 percent fat and not less than 8.25 percent non-fat milk solids (protein, milk sugar and minerals). It is generally fortified with vitamins D and A. Most fresh milk on the market is homogenized. Low-fat milk has a fat content that may vary between 0.5 and 2 percent, depending on state regulations.

Skim milk has virtually no fat—less than 0.5 percent and often as low as 0.1 percent (again, this varies from state to state). Do remember that skim milk has all the nutrients of whole milk except for the fat. Sometimes vitamins A and D are lacking, but skim milk is most often fortified with them.

Buttermilk is made by adding acid-producing bacteria to skim milk. It is much thicker than skim milk, but the fat content is the same.

Yogurt is also made by combining milk with a bacterial

culture. It may contain whole milk, but usually low-fat or skim milk is used.

Non-fat dry milk has all the nutrients of whole milk except the fat—provided that it is fortified with vitamins A and D.

Whole dry milk is also available.

Canned milk has been concentrated by removing part of the water. You can get either whole or skim canned milk. Sweetened condensed milk has sugar added to help preserve it.

Storage Fluid milk of any kind should be kept refrigerated in a covered container and used within a week.

Non-fat dry milk in an unopened package keeps at room temperature and should be used within a few months.

Dry whole milk should go into the refrigerator and should be used within a few weeks.

Evaporated milk should be stored at room temperature if unopened, and used within six months. If opened, cover and put in the refrigerator and use in three to five days.

As a general rule, favor the low-fat or non-fat milks or milk products. That way, you keep your consumption of saturated fats down. It's most healthful to stick with:

- Skim milk, in the container or dry
- Low-fat milk
- Buttermilk made from skim milk
- Yogurt made from skim or low-fat milk
- Cocoa made with skim milk
- Cheeses made from skim or low-fat milk (more about them later)

Remember the basics about milk fat: over half of it is saturated. Most of the remainder is monounsaturated—the fat that does not affect your cholesterol balance one way or the other. There is very little polyunsaturated fat. Think of whole milk as containing a fair amount of saturated fat per cup, and of cream as a concentrated source—so you really should go easy on cream. That does not mean you cannot have a small splurge now and then if you like it—your High Health diet gives you such a good safety margin.

Here is a table of the main fats in different milks and creams.

(The numbers do not add up to the total fat figure because some fatty acids that occur in very small proportions are omitted.)

Kind	Amount (1 cup) (gms.)	Total Fat (gms.)	Total Saturated Fatty Acids (gms.)	Unsaturated Fatty Acids Oleic (monounsaturated) (gms.)	Linoleic (polyunsaturated) (gms.)
Whole	244	8.5	4.7	2.8	.2
Low fat 2%	244	4.9	2.7	1.6	.1
Canned unsw.	252	19.9	10.9	6.6	.6
Condensed sw.	306	26.6	14.7	8.8	.8
Dry whole	128	35.2	19.4	11.6	1.0
Skim milk dry, +2% fat	250	5.8	3.2	1.9	.2
Plain skim milk	244	—	negligible		
Buttermilk (from skim milk)		—	negligible		
Human milk	244	9.6	4.8	3.2	.8
Cream, half 'n half 11.7% fat	242	28.3	15.6	9.3	.8
Cream, light 20.6% fat	240	49.4	27.2	16.3	1.5
Cream, heavy 37.6% fat	238	89.5	49.2	29.5	2.7

United States Department of Agriculture Publications

You will of course be saving quite a few calories by favoring the low-fat milks:

Whole milk	160 calories per cup
2% low-fat milk	130 calories per cup
1% low-fat milk	110 calories per cup
non-fat milk	90 calories per cup

Non-fat dry milk is generally a good buy, and you can use it not only to make skim milk, but mixed with dry ingredients in cooking or baking. Also, you can make a very good low-fat white sauce with skim milk. See the recipe on page 187.

CHEESES

Cheeses are a delicious and nourishing food, but most of them are quite high in saturated fat. Therefore, it is important to favor those made with skim or partially skimmed milk. When you do eat cheese made from whole milk, keep the portion small. Here is a good rule of thumb:

One ounce of whole-milk cheese contains roughly the amount of fat in an 8-oz. cup of whole milk.

The following table gives you a more detailed idea of just how much fat there is in some of the most common cheeses in this country:

Cheese	Amount	Total fat (gms.)	Total saturated fat (gms.)
Cream cheese	1 oz. (28 gms.)	10.7	5.9
Cheddar	"	9.1	5.0
Blue	"	8.6	4.8
Brick	"	8.6	4.8
Pimiento pasteurized process	"	8.6	4.7
American pasteurized process	"	8.5	4.7
Limburger	"	7.9	4.4
Swiss (domestic)	"	7.9	4.4
Swiss pasteurized process	"	7.6	4.2
Parmesan	"	7.4	4.1
Camembert	"	7.0	3.8
Cheese food, pasteurized processed American	"	6.8	3.7
Cheese spread, pasteurized processed American	"	6.1	3.3
Cottage cheese, dry curd with creamy mixture 4.2% milk fat		1.2	.7

United States Department of Agriculture Publications

You will have noticed that cottage cheese, even when creamed, is much lower in fat than the whole-milk cheeses in the table. Here are some other good low-fat cheeses to look for:

Uncreamed cottage cheese
Farmer's, hoop, or baker's cheese
Ricotta (made with partially skimmed milk)
Mozzarella (made with partially skimmed milk)
Sapsago
Processed cheeses made with skim milk and polyunsaturated

fats (various ones on, or coming on, the market). These are usually marked as cheese foods.

And how about

BUTTER?

Well, a good deal more than half of it is saturated. Then there is a fair amount of monounsaturated fat, and just a bit of polyunsaturate. So, as I have said, have a little butter if you like the taste, but go easy on it.

9

High Health Food Tips: Fish and Shellfish

Fish is a wonderful food. It is low in calories, it gives you first-rate protein, and although some fish contains a fair amount of fat, it is very polyunsaturated.

This means there are quite a few empty spaces where pairs of hydrogen atoms could hitch on. Most vegetable oils are not so polyunsaturated as this. In fact, fish takes the polyunsaturate prize as far as foods are concerned. There is scientific evidence that these very unsaturated oils are more effective than the lesser unsaturated ones in lowering the harmful kind of cholesterol in your blood.

How about dietary cholesterol? The levels in fish are very moderate. One study puts the average amount at about 70 milligrams per 100 grams—3½ ounces, an average serving. Fish with less fat contains less dietary cholesterol—something like 50 milligrams. On the other hand, canned sardines are on the high side in dietary cholesterol. So if you have a problem, that would be one product to restrict in your diet.

Fish are a low-calorie food in terms of their weight, but some varieties contain more fat than others. For most people this is nothing to worry about because of the excellent nature of the fat. However, if you are being very careful about your weight you may want to concentrate on the lower-fat fish.

Here is a list that should be helpful.

Fish with higher fat content

Herring
Mackerel
Pompano
Salmon (Atlantic and Chinook, either canned or raw)
Salmon (Sockeye)
Sardines (canned)
Shad
Trout (lake and rainbow)
Tuna (canned in oil)
Halibut (Greenland)

Fish with lower fat content

Bass (small mouth and large mouth)
Bluefish
Bullhead (black)
Catfish (freshwater)
Cod
Drum (freshwater)
Flounder
Haddock
Hake (whiting)
Halibut (Atlantic and Pacific)
Perch
Pike (walleyed)
Red and grey snapper
Red fish
Salmon (canned: Chum, Caho silver, Humpback [pink])
Salmon (raw: pink or smoked)
Sand dab
Sturgeon

Swordfish
Trout (brook)
Tuna (waterpack)
Whitefish

SHELLFISH

Shellfish have a reputation for being high in cholesterol, but recent studies indicate that this is not the case. The older methods of analysis mistook close cousins of cholesterol for cholesterol itself. Mussels, oysters, scallops, and clams are actually low-cholesterol foods, according to these revised estimates. Crab ranges from low to moderate. The only shellfish that tend toward higher cholesterol levels are shrimp and lobster. Given today's prices, you are not likely to consume huge amounts of these anyway.

Like fish, shellfish are excellent sources of protein.

BUYING FISH AND SHELLFISH

If you're buying fresh fish, be sure that it is absolutely fresh. You can gauge freshness by the non-fishy smell. Other things to watch for are rosy gills, stiff flesh, and bright eyes. Lobsters and crayfish should be alive when you buy them. The same goes for bivalves like oysters, clams, and mussels. The two shells must be tightly clamped together. Reject any with opened shells.

Fresh fish should be used right away. Chipped ice is the best way to keep fish if there is a delay between the time you buy it and the time you use it. The chipped ice prevents drying out.

Frozen fish and frozen shellfish are also very good. When thawing a package, leave it on a shelf in the refrigerator so that it defrosts slowly. Thawed fish loses its flavor very quickly, so be sure to cook it immediately. Never refreeze thawed fish.

COOKING FISH

There are many delicious ways to cook fish.

Here are a few brief notes:

Poaching: Prepare the court-bouillon—the seasoned fluid you do the poaching in—before you pour it over the fish. The court-bouillon doesn't take long—ten or fifteen minutes are enough, if you're a little pressed for time. Vinegar or lemon juice, onion, parsley, bay leaf, thyme, pepper and salt are classical ingredients. Be sure not to overcook fish. For instance, an average-size fillet of sole is done in three to five minutes. Simmer gently—don't boil.

Broiling: A good way to cook almost any fish. If it is very lean, like flounder, do it in a pan with just a touch of oil, to prevent sticking and give flavor. Try various seasonings like thyme, tarragon, dill, basil, rosemary.

Baking: A very good way to cook big fish. Use a little vegetable oil and seasoning.

Braising: Also very good for larger fish. But you will need a long fish kettle for best results. Covering the fish with aluminum foil in an ordinary pan is an alternative method.

Pan-frying: The modern no-stick pans are excellent for this cooking method as you need only a bit of oil or fat for flavoring. But you still do have to develop on your own the knack of turning the fish over with a spatula without breaking it.

10

High Health Food Tips: Oils and Margarines

About 40 percent of the fat in the average American diet comes from fats added to other foods—like butter, margarine, and cooking oils. These are the ones you can most easily control, naturally you want to make the right choices for a healthful diet.

As I have already said, you want to emphasize the vegetable oils because they have a beneficient effect on your cholesterol balance (when they are polyunsaturated) or at least do not change it the wrong way (when they are monounsaturated).

OILS

Let's have a look at those which are most widely available on the market, and which you may use in salads or in cooking. As with almost all fats, they are *mixtures* of unsaturated and saturated fatty acids, but the important point is that most of them are predominantly polyunsaturated.

If you look at the package labels you will notice that some refer to the "P/S" ratio. That is the proportion between the polyunsaturates and the saturates—and it is an important concept to bear in mind. (The monounsaturates are rarely if ever mentioned on the labels.) All oils, incidentally, have the same calorie content, which is about 120 for 1 tablespoon.

The oil with the highest P/S ration—in other words with the greatest amount of polyunsaturates compared to saturates—is safflower. It is approximately 10 to 1. That is why if a very special effort is being made to lower the harmful level of cholesterol, doctors will recommend that safflower oil be given first choice. Sunflower also has a high P/S.

Next comes corn oil, with a P/S ratio of 4 or 5 to 1. Then come soy oil with a P/S ratio of something over 3 to 1, sesame oil at 3 to 1, and cottonseed oil at about 2 to 1.

Peanut oil has a P/S ratio of about 5 to 3—but by now we have really gotten into a new group of oils, ones that have more monounsaturated fatty acids than either of the other two kinds. About half the content of peanut oil is monounsaturated.

Olive oil is the best example of the heavily monounsaturated oil—it is more than 75 percent monounsaturated. The saturate and polyunsaturate ingredients are roughly in balance.

Any one of these oils is good—certainly any is much better than the saturated fat which constitutes about two-thirds of the average American's fat consumption. If you wish to emphasize the polyunsaturate content, then choose an oil with one of the higher P/S ratings.

Just a reminder: Two vegetable oils are very saturated—palm kernel oil and coconut oil. They are rarely sold on the retail market, but you do find them in many commercial baked products and in a few margarines. It is best to avoid them as much as possible.

MARGARINES

They are made of one or more vegetable oils with some degree of processing. The key change to bear in mind is hydrogenation—the procedure I mentioned before which consists of adding hydrogen atoms to some of the empty spaces on the fatty acid chain. If the product is partially hydrogenated, that means it is less polyunsaturated than it was to begin with. If it is totally hydrogenated, then it is saturated. A vegetable oil that has been totally hydrogenated is no better for your health than a very saturated animal fat.

Margarines are often a mixture of two or more oils, and any one of these oils may have been subjected to the hydrogenation process.

As a general rule, the margarines you get in tubs are more polyunsaturated than the stick varieties. Most processors have started to put the P/S ratio on their labels, and it's a good idea to look at them. One survey showed that the highest P/S ratio, 7/2, was a soft margarine made up of some combination of cottonseed, safflower, sunflower and peanut oil. A few margarines had quite a low P/S ratio, 4/3.

Some margarines are more healthful for you than others. Since their composition may be changed from time to time it is important to study the labels on those available in your store.

Diet margarines These are simply margarines that have been diluted with water to reduce the calories—50 instead of 100 per tablespoon. The fact that a margarine is of the diet variety doesn't mean it has a better P/S rating.

Mayonnaise A lot of people think that mayonnaise is taboo in a careful diet. Actually, most mayonnaise has a good P/S ratio—two leading brands have ratios of 5/2 and 6/2. So mayonnaise can be like a good margarine. There is some dietary cholesterol if egg yolk is used, but it is an extremely small amount and nothing to worry about unless you have a special problem.

Other salad dressings They vary somewhat from product to product, but most have good P/S ratios, like 3 or 4 to 1.

Here is a table showing you the fat breakdown of some popular oils, margarines, and dressings.

Some Margarines, Oils, and Dressings

Content per Serving (1 tbsp., about 14 gms.)	Total Fat (gms.)	Poly-unsaturated (gms.)	Saturated (gms.)	Cholesterol (mg.)	Total Calories	Type of Oil
Margarines						
Blue Bonnet	11	4	3	0	100	soybean, cottonseed
Blue Bonnet (soft)	11	4	2	0	100	soybean, cottonseed
Chiffon (soft)	11	3	2	0	100	soybean
Fleischmann's (soft)	11	5	2	0	100	corn
Fleischmann's (diet)	6	2	1	0	50	corn
Imperial	11	3	3	0	100	soybean, palm
Imperial (soft)	11	4	3	0	100	soybean, palm
Mazola	11	3	2	0	100	corn, soybean, cottonseed
Mazola (diet)	6	2	1	0	50	corn
Mrs. Filberts Golden Quarters	11	1	2	0	100	soybean
Mrs. Filberts Golden (soft)	11	3	2	0	100	soybean
Mrs. Filberts Corn (soft)	11	5	2	0	100	corn
Mrs. Filberts (soft diet)	6	2	1	0	50	corn
Nucoa	11	3	2	0	100	soybean, cottonseed
Nucoa (soft)	10	3	2	0	90	soybean, cottonseed
Parkay (soft)	11	4	2	0	100	soybean
Promise	11	5	2	0	100	cottonseed, soybean safflower or sunflower
Promise (soft)	11	7	2	0	100	cottonseed, peanut, safflower or sunflower
Oils and Dressings						
Crisco Oil	14	5	2	0	120	soybean
Fleischmann's Corn Oil	14	8	2	0	120	corn
Kraft Safflower Oil	14	10	1	0	120	safflower
Mazola Oil	14	8	2	0	120	corn
Planter's Oil	14	5	3	0	126	peanut
Bright Day Imitation Mayonnaise	6	4	1	0	60	soybean and others
Hellmann's Real Mayonnaise	11	5	2	10	100	vegetable

Content per Serving (1 tbsp., about 14 gms.)	Total Fat (gms.)	Poly-unsat-urated (gms.)	Sat-urated (gms.)	Cholesterol (mg.)	Total Calories	Type of Oil
Oils and Dressings						
Kraft Real Mayonnaise	11	6	2	5	100	soybean
Mrs. Filberts Mayonnaise	11	6	2	10	100	soybean
Miracle Whip Salad Dressing	7	4	1	5	70	soybean
Mrs. Filberts Salad Dressing	6	3	1	10	65	soybean

From: *The Medical Letter*

11

How High Health Exercises Make Cholesterol Work for You

By now, I am sure you know exercise is good for your health, and in particular for your heart health. There have been many studies showing that people who exercise regularly tend to have less heart trouble. There is an especially revealing survey of thousands of Harvard graduates and what happened to them over the years. The more vigorously and regularly they exercised, the smaller were their chances of heart attack. The risk was only half as great in those expending 2000 calories in exercise per week (the equivalent of running a total of 20 miles at eight minutes per mile) compared to those who spent less than 500 calories.

Now we are finding out just what exercise does to blood cholesterol balances, which is such an important factor in cardiovascular health. Some very striking studies have been done by Dr. Peter D. Wood and his colleagues at the Stanford Heart Disease Prevention Program at Stanford University.

In one study, Dr. Wood took a group of dedicated runners and compared them to non-exercisers of similar age and background. The runners were middle-aged people—forty-five years old was the men's average, and forty-two the women's. They took their running seriously: the men averaged 37 miles a week, and the women 31.

It was no surprise to find that the runners were in much better shape than the non-runners. They had stronger hearts, their pulse rate at rest was lower, their blood pressure was lower, and they were leaner. In fact, their weight was approximately what it had been when they were eighteen.

CHOLESTEROL SHIFT

But the really fascinating finding of Dr. Wood was the difference in blood cholesterol. This wasn't very marked in the *total* cholesterol, although it was somewhat lower in the exercisers than in the non-exercisers. The big difference was in the *balance*.

The beneficial HDL cholesterol was much higher in the runners. Among the men, HDL averaged 64 for runners compared to 43 for non-runners. Among the women it was 75 compared to 56. HDL was about 50 percent higher in the people who exercised strenuously.

The harmful LDL cholesterol was lower in the runners: 125 instead of 139 for the men, and 113 instead of 123 for the women.

Some of the men runners actually had a cholesterol balance normally found only in young women. A few of the men, as well as a number of the women, actually had more HDL cholesterol than LDL cholesterol. This is extremely rare among adults, but is found in young children, various primitive peoples, and animals such as the rat or the dog, which have virtually no atherosclerosis.

Another interesting point was noticed: the blood triglyceride levels among the runners was only half of what it was among the sedentary volunteers.

Dr. Wood's experiments were of special interest because there were conflicting earlier reports about the effect of exercise on the *total* cholesterol level. Even if the total cholesterol does not change much, Dr. Wood showed, there is a very significant shift from the harmful to the helpful kind.

HOW ABOUT MODERATE EXERCISE?

What if you don't run 4 or 5 miles a day? Dr. Wood checked what happened following a moderate program of exercise for overweight women. It lasted seventeen weeks. Twice a week there was a twenty-minute session of walking/jogging, and twice a week a one-hour session of calisthenics and stretching exercises. The cholesterol changes were not so spectacular as the ones that occurred in the running enthusiasts. There was, however, a definite improvement in the HDL/LDL balance.

MARATHONERS, JOGGERS, SITTERS

Other reports confirm Dr. Wood's results. One recent study was conducted by G. Hartley Hartung, Ph.D., an authority on cardiac rehabilitation at Baylor College of Medicine in Houston.

Dr. Hartung studied three groups of middle-aged volunteers, all healthy professionals and businessmen. One group was made up of marathon runners who covered at least 40 miles a week. A second group was composed of people who jogged or ran 2 miles or so at least three times a week; few of these did more than a total of 20 miles a week. Finally there was the sedentary group—people who played golf a couple of times a week but did nothing sufficient to work up a sweat.

The study covered a five-month period, and the results were clear-cut: HDL levels were highest in the marathon runners, quite high in the joggers, and lowest in the non-exercisers. With total cholesterol, it went just the other way. Here is a tally of the findings:

	Mean Age	Total Cholesterol	HDL Cholesterol
59 marathon runners	44.5	187.2	64.8
85 joggers	46.8	204.2	58.0
74 sedentary men	46.1	211.7	44.3

Similarly, studies of more than 800 people done by Dr. John D. Cantwell and others at the Preventive Cardiology Clinic in Atlanta give a much higher HDL reading (average 58.5) to the physically fit than to the unfit (46).

SMOKING AND HDL

What besides diet and exercise affects your cholesterol balance? Recent studies are revealing some extremely significant information about smoking. A direct link has been made between cigarette smoking and HDL levels.

This has been one of the most striking findings in the so-called MR. FIT survey of 12,000 men in 20 U.S. cities over a six-year period. The letters stand for Multiple Risk Factor Intervention Trial. The purpose of MR. FIT is to find out how effective various life-style changes are in lowering the incidence of heart disease.

Smoking, it has been discovered, has a bad effect on blood cholesterol. Smokers have lower HDL levels than non-smokers. But if you quit, the MR. FIT findings show that your HDL is likely to rise.

There have been similar results in other studies, in particular a survey of almost 1000 men and women in Leiden, Holland.

The new knowledge about cholesterol seems to explain in part what we have known for a long time: that smoking is bad for your heart and your whole cardiovascular system. The more cigarettes a person smokes each day, and the longer they have had the habit, the greater their risk of cardiovascular disease.

Smoking is not only a direct cause of heart disease, but also has a number of indirect effects on the heart. For instance, it is the main cause of chronic bronchitis and emphysema, which are themselves the chief causes of pulmonary heart disease—and aggravate any kind of cardiovascular trouble.

People are much less aware of the heart dangers of smoking than they are of the cancer hazards. Actually, the heart toll of smoking is higher than the cancer toll. Look at it this way. It is estimated that 325,000 premature deaths a year are caused by cigarettes. Of this premature cigarette mortality, 19 percent comprises lung-cancer deaths, but about 37 percent are due to heart attacks. Smoking causes cancers other than lung cancer and other kinds of cardiovascular disease besides heart attacks, but these are the two main cigarette-caused killers.

In these days of soaring medical costs, you may be interested to know how much of them are attributable to smoking. The direct medical cost of cigarettes has been estimated at $8.2 billion per year in 1976 dollars. The total direct and indirect economic cost of smoking-induced diseases is over $27.5 billion.

But leaving these horrendous statistics and getting back to you as a person: If you happen to be a smoker, bear in mind the many studies that show your health risks will go down if you stop. Don't give up hope, just give up smoking.

I consider getting a patient to stop smoking as one of the most important things I can do for them. For instance, David F., fifty years old, a highly successful Baltimore businessman who had had a major heart attack four years before I saw him. He was still smoking the two packs a day he had become addicted to for the past thirty years. With proper management we were able to get him off this terrible habit. His HDL increased and there was also a smaller fall in his LDL. And his electrocardiogram became normal.

Alice J., forty-seven years old, was another heavy smoker who came to see me. She was an executive who had been told by her family doctor that she simply had to give up cigarettes as she had early signs of emphysema. Furthermore, her father had died of lung cancer, which suggested that there might be a family predisposition. Alice was eager to quit but besides the difficulty almost any smoker has in doing this, she was afraid of gaining weight. In talking to her, I stressed that even a big weight gain was nothing compared to cancer or emphysema—and also that there really is no need to gain weight when you stop smoking. She did give it up, and kept her weight down with diet and a good exercise program. Her blood profile showed a markedly lower LDL. HDL, which was already quite high, remained pretty much the same.

THE PILL

There has been much interest and some concern about the effect of the Pill on blood cholesterol. The Leiden study I mentioned earlier found that oral contraceptives were very much linked to lower HDL levels—and that this was particularly true for women who also smoked. However, other studies suggest that the Pill's effect on the cholesterol balance depends on its formulation. In one survey close to 5000 women taking oral contraceptives were checked. It was found that the HDL level went up with an increasing dose of estrogen, and went down when the progestin content of the Pill was increased. Women who used combinations of estrogens and progestins had HDL levels that were between those of estrogen users and those of progestin users.

There have been surveys indicating that most oral contraceptives lower HDL and increase LDL. We know that the Pill can be linked to thrombosis (blood clots) and other cardiovascular troubles, so a woman planning to go on the Pill would be wise to check her blood cholesterol before doing so, and then again a month or so after she has started. If her cholesterol balance has been adversely affected, her doctor may advise another formulation or a different method of birth control.

As a general rule caution is a must with the Pill if there are *any* heart risk factors such as—besides cholesterol—hypertension or a family history of cardiovascular trouble. And women on the Pill should make a point of not smoking.

I have found in my practice that an improved cholesterol

balance most often follows a woman's going off the Pill. This happened, for instance, with Faye M., twenty-three years old, a public relations person from Detroit. She had simply not been able to lose and keep off about 20 pounds that were very definitely surplus. I found that the Pill was causing her to retain excessive fluid. By changing to a different method of birth control, and with a moderate amount of dieting, Faye got down to a very good weight—and as an extra bonus raised her HDL and lowered her LDL.

OVERWEIGHT

If you are overweight and you reduce, you are likely to improve your cholesterol balance. That is one of the findings coming out of the MR. FIT study. There is a close link between increasing poundage and decreasing HDL. So you have one more reason to get rid of excess pounds.

Max S. was a forty-eight-year-old salesman who was concerned because he had gained 17 pounds during the previous four years—he was indulging in a few extra cocktails and rich desserts and was exercising less. Max had noticed that he was short of breath after climbing a single flight of stairs. This was of special concern to him because his brother had recently died of a heart attack. Tests also showed that he had an abnormally high LDL and a barely adequate level of HDL. I put Max on the reducing High Health Diet and the beginning phase of the High Health Exercise plan. In three months, he lost 16 pounds. His cholesterol balance showed a marked improvement. By then he had progressed to the more vigorous levels of the exercise plan, and his shortness of breath had entirely disappeared.

Another example is a woman from Virginia, Elizabeth T., forty-one years old. When she came to me she was 27 pounds overweight, and like so many of my patients had tried just about everything but with no lasting results. She had what I have called the Yo-Yo syndrome—she would lose weight and then gain it back again like a Yo-Yo going down and then back up. Elizabeth had problems metabolizing certain foods which I was able to correct, and with the proper diet and exercise got rid of her excess weight and kept it off. Her HDL reading was noticeably higher after she was down to normal weight.

LOSING POUNDS

In my practice, overweight is a problem I frequently have to deal with. And I have found that the High Health Diet (reducing version) is an excellent one for getting rid of unwanted pounds. One reason is that it is such a well-balanced regime that you get all the nutrients you need even at a fairly low calorie level.

To see just how well the reducing diet worked, I did a study covering several hundred patients. Here is a brief table showing the results:

Total number of patients studied: 580
Females: 379
Males: 201
Age range: six to ninety-three years of age
Average overweight before dieting: 18.3 pounds
Average weight loss per month: 9.7 pounds
Success: 407 patients (70 percent)
Failure: 173 patients (30 percent)

In most cases, the diet plus the right kind of exercise enabled the patient to get rid of excess weight and keep it off for at least six months. In a little less than a third of the cases, at first the diet was not successful. But with subsequent medical treatment plus the diet I was able to turn most of these failures around and make them successes. There were of course some adjustments of the diet for special cases, but the basic regime remained the High Health Diet.

I won't go into the medical aspects of the treatment here, but I would like to describe briefly a few of these cases, as that may be an encouragement to people with stubborn problems of overweight that may be linked to a medical condition. Of course if you have a medical problem, or suspect one, you should see your doctor and follow his or her advice about what to do. Don't go in for self-treatment:

Millie D., a fifty-six-year old woman from New Jersey, was 34 pounds overweight. After therapy, and with the diet, she was able to lose 31 pounds in a little over four months. This alleviated the pain from the arthritis from which she suffers.

Helen E., a twenty-four-year-old secretary, was 12 pounds overweight. This may not seem a lot, but it upset her a great deal. She had trouble reducing because she was so emotionally concerned about her acne. I sent her to a good dermatologist and then got her on a diet, and she lost six pounds in the first month.

Sue G. was eight pounds overweight. Her particular problem was very severe cramps before her menstrual period and also a craving for sweets at that time. We found she had an hormonal imbalance which we were able to correct. She then dieted successfully and lost 8 pounds in six weeks.

Wanda H., thirty-nine years old, from Kansas City, was 23 pounds overweight. Because of a thyroid dysfunction which had not been diagnosed, she was suffering from dry skin, brittle nails, loss of hair, and chronic fatigue. With medication we were able to correct her thyroid condition. Wanda then went on the diet and lost 17 pounds in three months.

Ted K., thirty-three years old, was 57 pounds overweight. He had a metabolic disturbance of hormonal origin which affected his sexual activity. This we were able to take care of. Ted then went on the reducing diet and lost 42 pounds. And he was still going down at that point.

Dick C., a twenty-seven-year-old dentist from Dallas, also had a metabolic disturbance that prevented him from burning calories properly. Besides his overweight, Dick was suffering from chronic fatigue and difficulty with many mental tasks. With treatment, the disorder was entirely cleared up. And with the diet, Dick got rid of his overweight, 21 pounds.

Betty was a twenty-eight-year-old telephone operator who came from Fort Worth, Texas. She was about 20 pounds too heavy. Most of the excess weight was in her trunk, particularly the back of her neck. Here, a hormonal imbalance was present. It was corrected with medication. Betty was then able to bring her weight down through dieting.

These are just a few cases among many. I want to stress again that I mention them simply to show that there is occasionally a medical condition that should be taken care of before dieting can succeed in taking off surplus pounds. Although, occasional, if it affects you, it is imperative that you get it corrected so you can take weight off, and keep it off permanently.

12

High Health Exercise Guidelines: Basics

Exercise has truly great benefits. It makes you look better. It makes you feel better and gives you the extra energy you want and need. And once you are in shape, you are able to deal with life's stresses much better.

As you increase your fitness, your heart gets stronger and more efficient. Each beat does more work, so your pulse at rest is lower than it was when you were out of condition. (Well-trained athletes often have resting pulse rates in the low fifties or the forties per minute.) Your blood pressure eases down to a lower, more healthful level. Your body, including your heart, uses oxygen more effectively. You develop more mitochondria, the tiny little basic power plants in each cell.

I've already mentioned the very healthful cholesterol balance (higher HDL, lower LDL) that vigorous exercise brings. There are other benefits, too. Vigorous exercise may reduce blood triglycerides, which can be a risk if their level is too high. And in a fit body the blood has less tendency to clot—

so there's less change of blockage that causes stroke and heart attack.

Furthermore, as you get into shape, your body composition changes. The proportion of body fat goes down and lean muscle mass goes up. Before you know it, you may be back to trim twenty-year-old standards—12 to 13 percent body fat for men, 25 percent for women.

If you are trying to lose weight, I can assure you that exercise should be an integral part of your regime—along with the right diet. You will lose weight more easily and more healthfully that way. Think of exercise and diet as partners.

THE THREE KINDS OF EXERCISE

There are three main kinds of exercise, and you should do all three to achieve real fitness and high health.

First there is exercise that makes and keeps you limber, that prevents muscles from shortening, that maintains the fullest range of joint movement, like touching your toes. This kind is usually called *stretching* or *flexibility* exercise.

Then there is *strengthening* exercise which builds up the power of various skeletal muscles. Push-ups are a good example.

Last, but definitely not least, comes exercise that conditions your heart-lung system: *endurance* or *aerobic* exercise. What this does is improve your ability to take in oxygen, send it all around your body in your blood thanks to the heart's pumping action, and use it in the production of energy.

Endurance exercise is the most important. It is the only way to get your cardiovascular system in good condition. It requires using the big muscles of your body in a steady, rhythmical way so that you raise your heartbeat and your rate of breathing. Fast walking, jogging or running, vigorous swimming, cross-country skiing, rowing, aerobic dancing, and jazz exercise are excellent. So are sports like squash and racquet ball. And tennis, if you really keep going.

To be effective, endurance activity has to be done continuously over a period of time. A sensible minimum to shoot for is twenty minutes three times a week. Of course, if you're out of shape you'll have to build up to this gradually. More about that later.

WARM-UP AND COOL-DOWN

Your endurance workout should be preceded by a brief warm-up—at least five minutes—and followed by a cool-down of the same length. You can work some limbering exercises into these periods and two or three strengthening exercises if you like.

The warm-up has several purposes. It gets your muscles and your joints ready for the vigorous exercise that lies ahead. A "cold" muscle isn't so supple as a warm one and is therefore more easily injured. Also, it is best to get your heartbeat up gradually because a sudden load put on it might be dangerous if you are not in good condition.

The cool-down is also important. If you stop abruptly after strenuous exercise, the blood that has been coursing through your muscles slows down and may be trapped for a moment. As a result your brain may not get enough and you will feel faint or dizzy. Or your heart muscle won't get sufficient blood, in which case you may notice some extra heartbeats. If your intestines are deprived of blood, you will probably feel nauseated.

The cool-down enables you to reduce your blood pressure and pulse rate smoothly and gradually. You may have noticed athletes cooling down with slow jogging or walking, or horses getting walked after a race. It's important to follow their example.

HOW OFTEN?

It is best to make exercise a daily habit, but if you can't manage this, try to get in at least three periods of endurance exercise a week, and an equal number of stretching and strengthening sessions.

START SLOWLY

If you haven't been doing much except getting to the office or driving to the shopping center, be sure to start your exercise program slowly and increase it gradually over the weeks and months. I find that the simplest and most practical way to get sedentary patients started is plain walking. More about that in the next chapter.

MAKING PROGRESS

Soon after you start your exercise program you will notice you feel better—and after three or four weeks you will observe a very definite improvement in the distance you cover or the speed. In two or three months, you will be quite a new person. And from then on to perhaps five or six months from the start of your program you may reach a peak level.

Always remember these two key principles:

1. Don't force yourself. Don't try to rush ahead. Don't compete with other people—or with what you did yesterday.

2. As you shape up, you will find that you have to increase your exertion level to get your heartbeat up into the training range. In other words, what represents a good healthy effort when you start out will get to be too easy after a while.

You will find more detailed advice in the next two chapters.

MEDICAL CHECKUP

It is a good idea to check with your doctor before launching into an exercise program. If you are in your twenties or early thirties, are in pretty good condition, and have never had any serious medical problem, you may not need a physical examination. But it is certainly advisable if you are over thirty-five and have not been very active recently.

If you have—or have had—any problem such as heart trouble you should be sure to consult your doctor before starting no matter what your age. That does not mean vigorous exercise is ruled out—exercise is now used routinely in the rehabilitation of people who have had heart attacks, and some of them after a long and very gradual buildup have gone on to marathon running. But you should follow a program that has your doctor's okay.

Here is a checklist. If your answer to any of these questions is yes, be *sure* to see your doctor before starting your program.

- Has anything ever been wrong with your heart?
- Do you ever get a pain in your chest when you exercise? Going up stairs? Or in a cold wind?
- Do you ever have spells of rapid or irregular heartbeats?
- Has there been much heart trouble among your blood relatives?
- Did you have rheumatic fever as a child?
- Do you have high blood pressure? Or did you in the past?
- Are you a heavy smoker?
- Are you very much overweight—say, 20 to 25 pounds?
- Do you have diabetes?
- Do you have emphysema or any other lung disorder?
- Do you have asthma?
- Do you have arthritis? Any problems with your joints? With your back? Your legs? Your feet?
- Do you get cramps in your legs after walking a short distance?
- Have you had any liver trouble?
- Is anything wrong with your kidneys?
- Are you severely anemic?
- Do you have any chronic sickness?
- Are you taking any medication regularly?

I want to stress again that a "yes" answer to any of these questions does not necessarily mean you cannot undertake an exercise program. You may simply have to be more careful at first, or take one or two simple precautions. The way to determine this is with your doctor.

SPECIAL CARE

People with certain disorders should exercise only in a medically supervised rehabilitation program. The American Medical Association mentions in particular the following conditions:

A heart attack after two months
Angina pectoris
Moderate to severe hypertension
Massive obesity
Severe arthritis or other major troubles affecting bones or muscles
Severe varicose veins
Any recent bleeding problems

Also requiring special precautions are poorly controlled convulsive disorders, multiple sclerosis, and peripheral vascular disease.

NO

There are a few conditions that do rule out participation in an exercise program. They include:

A *recent* heart attack
Changing patterns of angina
Severely damaged heart valves
Certain heart irregularities
Severe obstructive lung disease
Uncontrolled diabetes
Uncontrolled hypertension

Severe anemia
Acute infectious disease

Anyone in these categories should be under a doctor's care.

WARNING SIGNS AND WHAT TO DO

When you take up systematic exercise, know your warning signs. If any of the following happens during or after exercising, stop your program and check with your doctor before resuming it—or immediately if the symptoms persist at all.

1. Pain in the chest or radiating into the throat or arms. This is not necessarily a sign of heart trouble, but it could be. (Regardless of exercise, if you ever have these symptoms for more than a minute or two, get to a hospital emergency room.)

2. Irregular heartbeats—palpitations, or a series of abnormally fast or slow beats. These kinds of irregularities can be harmless. Or they may require medical attention. Continued fast pulse five or ten minutes after exercising may mean you have been pushing yourself too hard.

3. Dizziness, cold sweat, confusion. This probably means your brain is not getting enough blood. First aid: Lie down and put your feet up.

Some other points:

- Nausea after exercise, prolonged fatigue, insomnia, indicate you are exercising too vigorously.
- If you have any arthritic or other joint problems that flare up, you may know from past experience how to deal with them. If they persist or get worse, check with your doctor.
- Shin splints and other muscular aches and pains are very often helped by shoes with thicker soles. If necessary shift to another exercise—for instance biking instead of jogging—until the ailment clears up.

DOS AND DON'TS

Here is some additional advice from AMA experts about stretching and strengthening exercise:

- Avoid jerky movements. Use full rhythmic ones instead.
- In general, don't do more than fifteen or twenty consecutive repeats of an exercise affecting one muscle group during one period.
- Don't rush through limbering and strengthening exercises. Take minibreaks—especially if you are just starting.
- Be sure to exercise your abdominal muscles. They are often weak.
- Be very careful with isometric exercises. Especially . . .
- Don't hold your breath while doing them—or any other exercise.
- If you don't have a good mat, avoid kneeling or rolling-on-your-back exercises. Or do them on your bed.
- Don't bounce when you are doing limbering exercises (the static, straining kind). Just stretch a little, gently.
- Don't overwork one muscle or group of muscles.
- Don't do bending exercises with your knees locked.
- And before you do them, do sideways bending.
- Avoid alcohol during a three-hour period before exercising.

P.S. Don't let any of these cautions scare you off from a good exercise regime. Just bear them in mind to avoid getting into trouble.

13

The High Health Exercise Plan: How to Get Going

Let's assume that you have been getting little or no exercise for quite a long time. Your problem is how to get started in a safe and effective way.

The first question you should ask yourself is do you need a medical check first? If you are in doubt about this, pick up the phone and ask your doctor. If you don't have a family doctor, this is a good time to get one.

Your doctor may be able to do all the checks he believes necessary himself—like blood pressure, blood analysis, a bench-stepping test, and an electrocardiogram. He may also suggest that you have an exercise stress test at a specialized center.

STRESS TEST

These special tests monitor your heart and lung action as you exercise harder and harder on a treadmill or a stationary bicycle. Many experts feel they are extremely useful. They believe stress-testing gives a much better reading of a person's physical fitness and that it can also reveal hidden heart risks in persons who seem to be in excellent condition.

However, some studies indicate that stress tests may give quite a few "false-positive" and "false-negative" results—in other words, results indicating that something is wrong when it is not, or that everything is all right when in fact something is wrong. This can bring about unwarranted anxiety in the first case and a false sense of security in the second.

In any case, if your doctor feels you should have a stress EKG, you should follow the advice. In properly given stress tests, incidentally, qualified personnel should always be present in case the person being tested is pushed just a little too hard and needs emergency care. This happens in only a very small number of cases. Modern emergency aid will virtually always be successful in such an event, and no permanent harm is likely. And valuable information leading to the right treatment has been acquired. If a person has had any history of heart trouble, a doctor should be present at the stress test.

Stress tests do cost money, and facilities are not always available. Consequently, most people get into exercise programs without a stress test. A very famous Swedish authority, Per Olof Astrand, has remarked that the people who really need a test are those who risk their health by not exercising.

DO-IT-YOURSELF FITNESS TESTS

There are a number of simple tests that may give a person an idea of how fit he is—such as seeing how fast your heart beats after stepping up and down on a bench for a certain number of minutes, or how far you can run in a given time. The trouble with many of these is that they present some risk to the layman who is in poor or even fair shape. They inevitably push him or her to some degree or there would not be any testing effect, and the self-tester may not be aware that he is overexerting. Unless you know you are in good shape and just want to see how you measure up, I would be very cautious about these do-it-yourself tests.

There are, however, one or two very simple tests that can be done without undue risk. Here is one recommended for beginners by the President's Council of Physical Fitness and Sports.

THE BEGINNER'S WALK TEST

See how many minutes up to a maximum of ten you can walk at a brisk pace on a level surface without discomfort or difficulty. "Brisk" here simply means what seems brisk to you. If there is any discomfort or difficulty, you should stop, or at least slow down.

If you cannot walk briskly for five minutes, that puts you into the lowest of three beginner categories.

If you can walk briskly for more than five minutes but less than ten, that puts you into a middle beginner's category.

If you can breeze through ten minutes' of brisk walking, then you are in an upper beginner's category.

A more sophisticated do-it-yourself test has been worked out by Fred Kasch, Ph.D., of San Diego State University. All it requires is a bench twelve inches high (a pile of newspapers, magazines, or big books tied together works), and a watch with a second hand.

Here is how it goes:

- Step up and down at the rate of 24 round trips per minute—that is 2 up-and-downs every five seconds.
- Do this for three minutes.

- Sit down immediately and relax.
- Five seconds later start taking your pulse.
- Take it for sixty seconds—1 full minute.

This is a quite moderate level of exertion, and should not be too difficult for most people. However, if at any time you feel that you are straining, STOP IMMEDIATELY and list your fitness as poor. DON'T take the test without medical advice if you have any history of heart trouble or any serious health problem.

You can find your pulse not only at the traditional wrist point, but at your temple, at the side of your neck, at your groin, and a number of other spots. Do whatever is easiest.

To find out your fitness level, see where your after-test pulse rate is on the following chart. If your age group is not on it, use the closest age figure.

Fitness	6-12 yrs.		18-26 yrs.		33-57 yrs.	
Level	Boys	Girls	Men	Women	Men	Women
Excellent	73-82	81-92	69-75	76-84	63-76	73-86
Good	83-92	93-104	76-83	85-94	77-90	87-100
Average	93-103	105-118	84-92	95-105	91-106	101-117
Fair	104-113	119-130	93-99	106-116	107-120	118-130
Poor	114-123	131-142	100-106	117-127	121-134	131-144

PULSE-RATE YOURSELF

Exercise for a couple of minutes and then stop and take your pulse. (A couple of fingers on your temple is an easy way if you have trouble finding your wrist pulse.) Count your heart-beats for ten seconds and then multiply by six to get the rate per minute. You can't get a good readout if you take much longer than that, because your heart starts slowing down almost immediately.

Your goal is to get your heart rate up to 70 to 85 percent of its maximum rate. This varies from person to person. It depends on your condition and your age. As you get older, your maximum heart rate goes down.

One formula for figuring out your maximum rate is to subtract your age from 220. For a person who is twenty, it would be about 200, for a person who is thirty it would be about 190 and so on.

The target exercise rate for a young person of twenty would be 75 percent of 200, in other words about 150. For someone forty years old, the maximum would be approximately 180, and 75 percent of that is 135. Here is what it looks like on a chart.

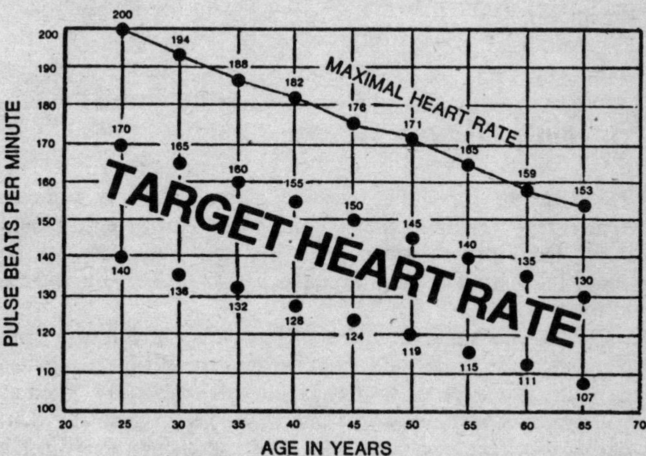

You will notice that the target zone for training provides not only something to aim for but also tells you what not to go beyond. As a rule you never want to go beyond that 85 percent level unless you are really in top condition. During the beginning part of your exercise program, don't go much above the lower 70 percent level at any time.

If your heart rate is not up to the 70 percent training level, then try exercising just a little harder for a minute or so and see if you can reach it.

After a while, you will get to know instinctively if you are in the target range. It is exercise that gives you a definite feeling of exertion, that causes you to breathe faster and perhaps perspire. But it is *not* anything like an all-out effort.

One easy way to see if you are in the training range and not above it is the talk test. If you can carry on a conversation with someone—say a jogging companion—you are probably not overexerting. If you are too breathless to talk, then you are overdoing it.

If you are an out-of-shape beginner, I would not worry too much at first about raising your pulse to the target zone. Just get going *easily,* and keep on your beginner's program until you have gotten somewhere.

THE BIG THREE QUESTIONS

There are three essential questions about endurance exercise at any stage, including the beginning one: How intense should it be? How long should it last? And how often should it be done? Intensity. Duration. Frequency. Always keep those three in mind.

When you start, all three will be low. If you're a rank beginner, just some mild exercise for ten or fifteen minutes three times a week or so may be all you want to do. Then as you progress week by week, intensity goes up gradually. Duration also increases. And instead of exercising three times a week you may be doing it five or six times a week, or even every day.

The important thing is to progress *slowly,* not to push yourself to the point of discomfort, and not to try to meet some rigid standard or to do better than you did the day before.

THE SUIT-YOURSELF STARTER PROGRAM

There is no single "best" endurance exercise for everyone, but the easiest and most practical one for most people is plain walking.

You can have a very flexible program, or you can have one with more structure. Here is an excellent way to start a flexible one:

Figure out a walk that is a mile long. You can do this by counting city blocks if they are regular (like 20 to a mile going north-south in New York City) or by measuring a mile stretch along a road with your car's odometer.

Start walking a little every other day and then every day until you are up to walking 1 mile. Let's say it takes you twenty-five or thirty minutes—a slow walk.

Now start walking just a little faster—always keeping it entirely comfortable—until you are covering that same mile in twenty minutes. It may take you three or four days to get up to this speed. Or it may take you a couple of weeks. It doesn't matter.

One mile in twenty minutes is a fairly good walking speed. Keep doing the twenty-minute mile daily until you are absolutely easy with it.

Now start lengthening your walk while keeping at the same speed, until you reach the level of 2 miles in forty minutes.

Again, stay at this level until it is perfectly comfortable.

Now keep the 2-mile distance but start walking a little faster—until you are covering the 2 miles in thirty minutes. That is 4 miles an hour—a very respectable clip. It may take you quite some time to go from forty minutes to thirty minutes for your 2-mile walk. Be sure to take all the time you need.

Once again, keep at this level—2 miles in thirty minutes—for a while, until it is easy.

Then start lengthening your walk again without changing your speed until you are covering 3 miles in forty-five minutes.

By this time you are no longer a beginner. It may take you three or four weeks to reach the 3-miles-in-forty-five-minutes level. Or it may take you a couple of months—or more. Always remember the principle: Go at your own pace. And increase your pace at your own rate.

You may now continue your walking program in the same way, aiming at the very vigorous walking rates of 4 ½ or even 5 miles per hour, or lengthening your walk to one hour, or both.

WANT A LITTLE MORE STRUCTURE?

Some people like a more specific program to follow. If you do, here is the beginner's walking program worked out by experts of the President's Council.

- First, take the beginner's walk test I described earlier.
- If you can't walk briskly for five minutes, begin the Red Walking Program (which follows) at the start—with the first week.
- If you can walk briskly more than five minutes, but less than ten, begin the Red Walking Program at the third week.
- If you can do the full brisk ten-minute walk but feel a little tired and sore, start with the first week of the White Walk–Jog Program (which follows).
- If you can breeze through the ten-minute walk, start with the third week of the White Walk–Jog Program.
- If you want to stick to walking throughout, just substitute fast walking for jogging.

BEGINNER'S RED WALKING PROGRAM

First week: Walk briskly for five minutes, or less if it is uncomfortable. Then walk slowly or rest for three minutes. Then walk briskly again for five minutes—or until you are uncomfortably tired. Walk every other day.

Second week: Follow the same routine as the first week but increase your pace as soon as you can walk five minutes without fatigue or soreness. (Walk every other day.)

Third week: Walk at a brisk pace for eight minutes, or for a shorter time if you become uncomfortably tired. Walk slowly or rest for three minutes. Again, walk briskly for eight minutes or until you are tired. (Walk four times a week.)

Fourth week: Follow the same routine as the third week, but increase the pace as soon as you can walk eight minutes without fatigue or soreness. (Walk five times a week.)

When you have completed the fourth week you may go on to the White Walk–Jog Program. (Substitute fast walking for jogging if you want to stick to an all-walking plan.)

The White Walk–Jog Program

Note: Walk-jog or fast-walk/walk exercise four times a week.

First week: Walk briskly for ten minutes, or less if you become uncomfortable. Walk slowly for three minutes. Then walk briskly again for ten minutes, or less if you become uncomfortable.

Second week: Walk briskly for fifteen minutes, or less if you become uncomfortable. Then walk slowly for three minutes.

Third week: Jog ten seconds (about twenty-five yards). Walk one minute (a hundred yards). Do twelve times.

Fourth week: Jog twenty seconds (fifty yards). Walk one minute (a hundred yards). Do twelve times.

When you have finished the four weeks of The White Walk–Jog Program, you are ready to start at the first week of The Blue Jogging Program. Again, if you prefer, substitute *fast* walking for the jogging—and use the same schedule.

The Blue Jogging Program

Note: Exercise five times a week throughout the eight-week program.

First week: Jog forty seconds (a hundred yards). Walk one minute (a hundred yards). Repeat nine times.

Second week: Jog one minute (a hundred fifty yards). Walk one minute (a hundred yards). Do eight times.

Third week: Jog two minutes (three hundred yards). Walk one minute (a hundred yards). Do six times.

Fourth week: Jog four minutes (six hundred yards). Walk one minute (a hundred yards). Do four times.

Fifth week: Jog six minutes (nine hundred yards). Walk one minute (a hundred yards). Do three times.

Sixth week: Jog eight minutes (twelve hundred yards). Walk two minutes (two hundred yards). Do twice.

Seventh week: Jog ten minutes (fifteen hundred yards). Walk two minutes (two hundred yards). Do twice.

Eighth week: Jog twelve minutes (seventeen hundred and sixty yards—or a mile). Walk two minutes (two hundred yards). Do twice.

This concludes the beginner's program. I'll have some suggestions about carrying on from here in the next chapter.

A NOTE ABOUT WALKING

Jogging and running are of course excellent endurance exercises, but they are not for everyone. The continuous jolting may be harmful to people with weak feet, knees, or hips. Walking, on the other hand, has much less wear and tear, because both feet are never off the ground simultaneously. People who are overweight or who have joint problems are better off walking.

Another advantage of walking, especially for beginners, is that there is virtually no risk of overstressing your heart.

Do not underestimate the amount of exercise you can get with the walk. Walking at four miles an hour is real exercise and has a very definite training effect on your cardio-pulmonary system. And if—after getting into good shape—you can push up to 4½ or even 5 miles an hour, you will understand why walking is an Olympic sport.

MAKING PROGRESS: ENDURANCE

As you build up your endurance you will find that a given intensity of exercise is not enough to bring your pulse into the training range. So it is a good idea to pulse-test yourself periodically to see how you are doing. Or, as I mentioned previously, you may have developed an instinctive way of sensing if you are at a satisfactory level, and of pushing yourself just a little harder when something gets a little bit too easy.

Here are some basic stretching and strengthening exercises that are good for any exercise program. Include at least half-a-dozen of each group in your daily exercise routine. After them I'll have some suggestions about endurance activities that can fit easily into your life.

14

The High Health Exercise Plan: How to Keep at It

Once you are past the beginner's stage, your endurance activity should be at least twenty minutes at your training level. It should be preceded and followed by a warm-up and a cool-down of at least five minutes each.

Although endurance exercise is the most important kind, stretching and strengthening are also essential. Stretching exercises keep you limber and lessen the chance of muscle or tendon tears. And they enable you to avoid the muscular tightening-up that happens in your body with various forms of strenuous exertion. For instance, if you run there are three or four stretching exercises that are absolutely essential.

Strengthening exercises are also important. They build up support for your joints. They balance muscles you use a lot by exercising their opposite numbers, the antagonists. They get you into better shape for sports.

You can use the warm-up and cool-down periods for stretching exercises. You can also work in strengthening exercises during these two periods if you wish. However, the warm-up should also include some aerobic exercise, like slow jogging before running. And the cool-down should always have some easy moving around, such as walking a few minutes after a run.

BASIC EXERCISE PACKAGE

So your basic exercise routine goes:

- Five minutes or more of warm-up, including some stretching and strengthening
- Twenty minutes or more of endurance activity
- Five minutes or more of cool-down, including some stretching or strengthening.

This should be done at least three times a week. Four or five times is better, but the three-per-week schedule will give you results—and keep you in shape once you have achieved the desired fitness level. Some people like to have a good endurance workout three times a week, and use the alternate days for twenty or thirty minutes of stretching and strengthening calisthenics.

It is ideal to work different sports into your program. Try to have four or five you can play depending on the season, where you are, and what the weather is doing. For example, you might include tennis, hiking, skiing, dancing, and swimming.

Just about any sport does good things to you and makes a

major contribution to your fitness. However, only a few have the *sustained* endurance activity you need if you want to become aerobically fit. For instance, a top-notch tennis player playing at a fast clip with very few breaks may very well be getting as much of an endurance workout as a runner. But very few amateur players get up to this level.

As a general rule, remember you have to be fit *before* you go in for strenuous sports. If you want to play squash you have to be in top cardio-pulmonary condition or you may get into serious trouble. Even professional tennis players build up their endurance with complementary activities like running.

FLEXIBILITY TESTS

It's a very good idea to find out how flexible you are and there are a few simple tests that will help you do this. Here they are:

Bend your left thumb back toward your forearm with your right hand (or the other way around). If you can get it all the way back, you are probably extremely loose-jointed. If you can't get your thumb back beyond a right angle, you are probably tight-jointed. The further back you can get your thumb, the looser you are.

Keep your legs straight and see if you can touch the ground with your palms. (Don't force.) If your palms touch, you are very flexible. If you cannot touch the ground at all, even with your fingertips, you are on the tight side.

When you stand with your knees straight and tensed, do they bend back slightly? If so, you are probably flexible all over.

When you straighten out an arm horizontally with the palm of your hand up, does your forearm go a little beyond a straight line and bend down slightly? Another sign of flexibility.

If you are tight, you are more liable to pull or even tear a muscle or tendon when you are physically active. So you should emphasize stretching exercises more than the strengthening ones.

If you are loose, you run a greater risk of spraining various joints—the knees are particularly vulnerable. So you want to emphasize exercises that strengthen muscles and tendons that give bracing and support to joints.

STRENGTH TESTS

There are some home tests you use to rate the strength of important muscular areas. See if you can do each of the following strengthening exercises just once (you will find them in the exercises section a little further on):

- Situp—the easiest version, with your arms at your side
- Leg lift
- Back raise
- Push-up

According to Dr. Hans Kraus, who developed these tests, not being able to do each exercise at least once indicates a very low level of strength which should be corrected.

MAKING PROGRESS: STRETCHING AND STRENGTHENING

In the stretching and strengthening exercises which follow, I have indicated a certain number of repetitions for each. That does not mean you start off at that level—at the beginning, just do one or two, or whatever is easy. Increase the number as you go along, again following the principle of comfortable progression. You may also want to increase the repetitions beyond the suggested number once you are in good shape.

In general, it is sufficient to allow about one minute for one exercise. Some may take less, some more.

Remember the very important point about stretching: *don't force yourself*. And don't do that bobbing and bouncing that used to be the fashion. It is harmful to ligaments and muscles. Think of stretching as easy and static rather than dynamic.

Here are some basic stretching and strengthening exercises that are good for any exercise program. Include at least half-a-dozen of each group in your daily exercise routine. After them I'll have some suggestions about endurance activities that can fit easily into your life.

STRETCHING EXERCISES

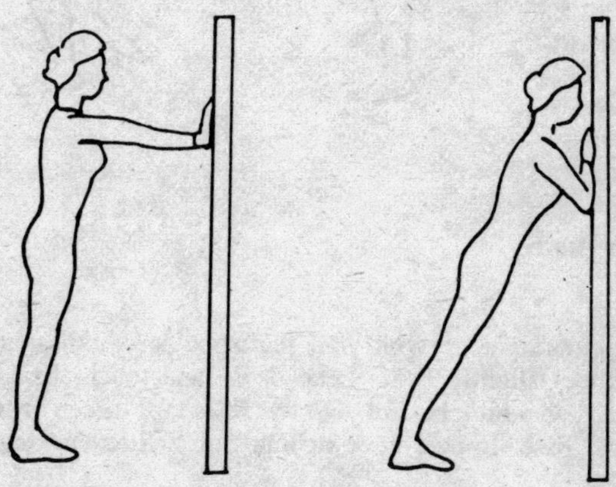

PUSH-IN

Stand three feet from the wall, straight, with palms on wall. Let yourself into wall, keeping your feet flat on the ground. You will feel a stretch in your calves. Hold fifteen seconds. Repeat four times. You can increase the stretching effect by moving farther from wall. Stretches calf muscles and Achilles tendon.

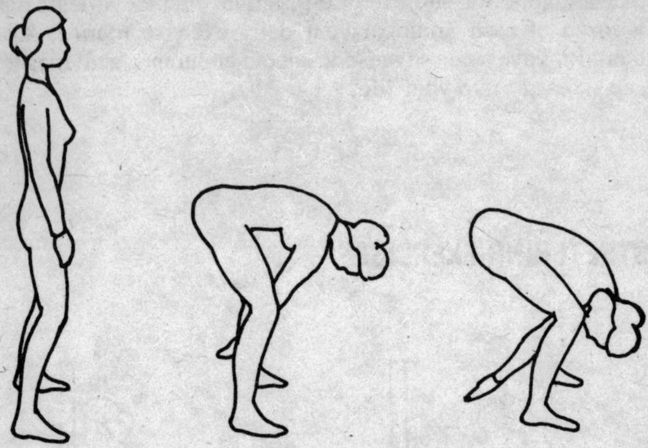

Front Bend

Stand straight up with your feet shoulder-width apart and your knees slightly bent. Lean down and touch the ground between and a little behind your feet. Hold for fifteen or twenty seconds. Rise. Repeat three or four times. Stretches legs and back.

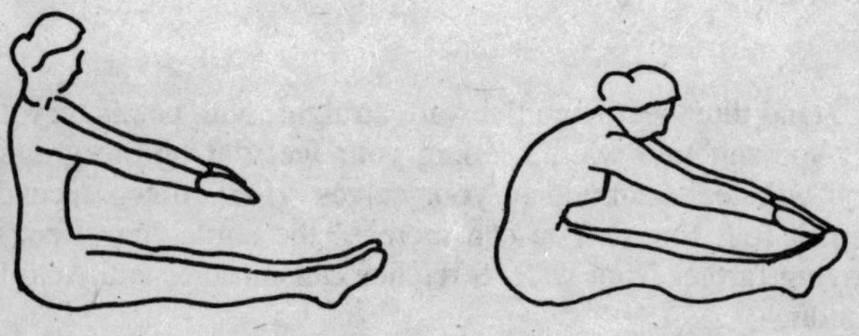

Toe Touch

Sit on ground with legs in front of you and arms stretched out in front. Lean forward as far as possible and grasp ankles. Pull yourself gently a little farther. Hold ten seconds. Relax. Repeat five times. Stretches back and hamstrings (the muscles in the back of your thigh).

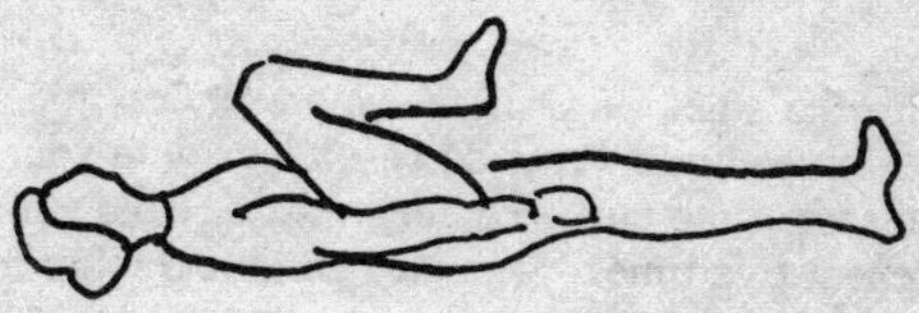

Knee Pull

Lie flat on your back. Raise one knee up and pull it toward your chest as far as comfortable. Hold four or five seconds. Repeat six or eight times with each leg. Stretches thigh and trunk muscles.

Important note: Any exercise that has you lie on your back requires a good thick exercise pad or carpet if you want to lie on the floor. Otherwise, do it on your bed. You can hurt your back if you do any kind of rolling motion lying on it against a hard surface.

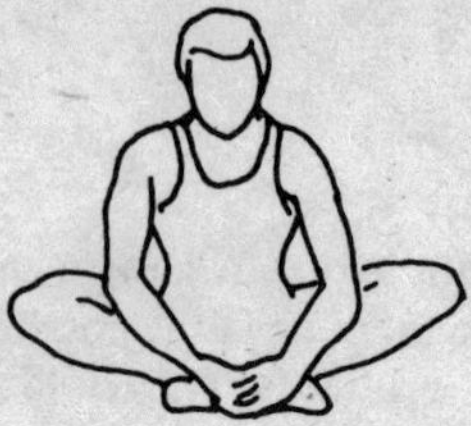

TOE PULL

Sit with the soles of your feet more or less together and your knees spread out. Press down on legs with your elbows, and at the same time pull your feet inward. Hold ten seconds. Relax. Repeat five times. Stretches groin and thigh muscles.

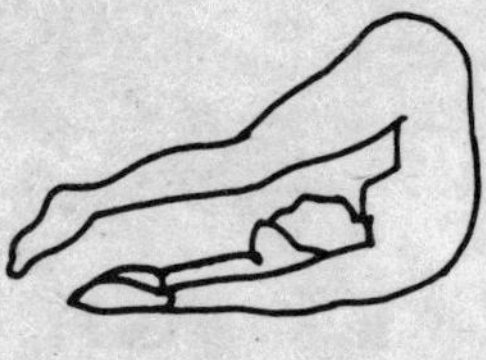

BACKOVER (Avoid if you have had any trouble with your neck or back.)

Lie on back with arms stretched out flat above your head. Bring your legs over your head and down toward the floor as far as you can go comfortably. Hold for ten seconds. Relax. Repeat five times. Stretches back of thigh (hamstrings) and lower back. Fairly advanced.

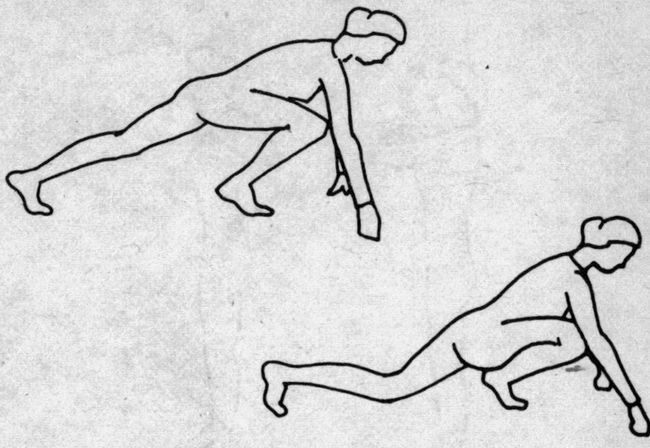

STRIDE STRETCH

Take the position of a sprinter at the starting line, one leg stretched back, the other flexed forward, hands on floor in front. Hold five seconds. Relax. Do other leg. Repeat six times each leg. Stretches groin and leg muscles.

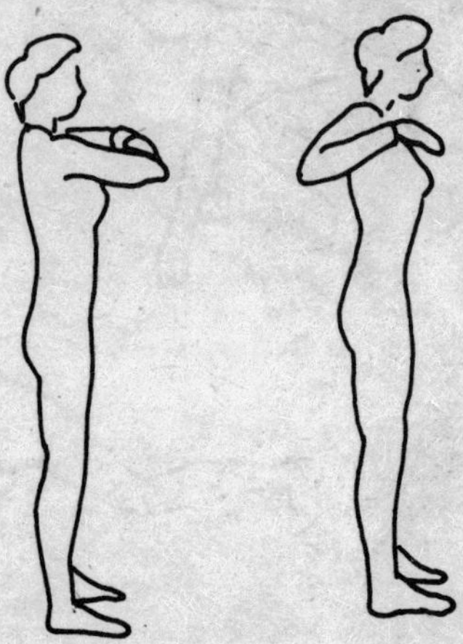

WINGING

Feet apart, standing straight, arms bent and parallel to the ground, elbows out to side. Thrust elbows back, then return to starting position. Repeat ten or fifteen times. Stretches shoulder and back muscles.

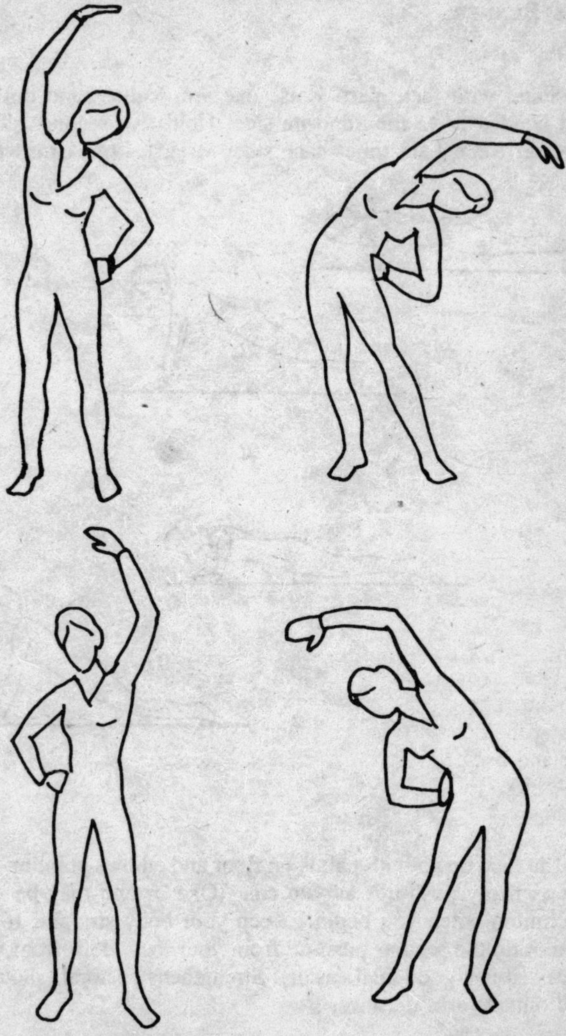

SIDE BENDER

Stand with feet apart. Raise one arm (other hand on hip) and bend over to the opposite side. Hold five seconds. Then reverse. Repeat six times each side. Stretches trunk muscles.

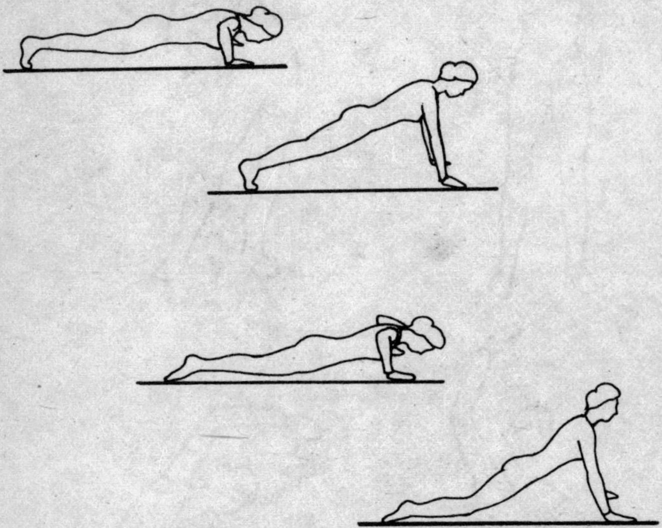

PUSH-UP

Lie face down with palms on floor and elbows pointing out. Do as many push-ups as you can. (One or two may be your maximum when you begin.) Keep your body straight. If you cannot do the regular push-up from your toes, do it from your knees (it is a good deal easier). Strengthens pectoral, shoulder and outside arm muscles.

Situps

The most important single strengthening exercise you can do is the one for your abdomen, which doesn't get used very strenuously in most sports. A firm belly is essential for good posture and for protection against the lower-back trouble that plagues so many millions of Americans. Here are some of the basic exercises.

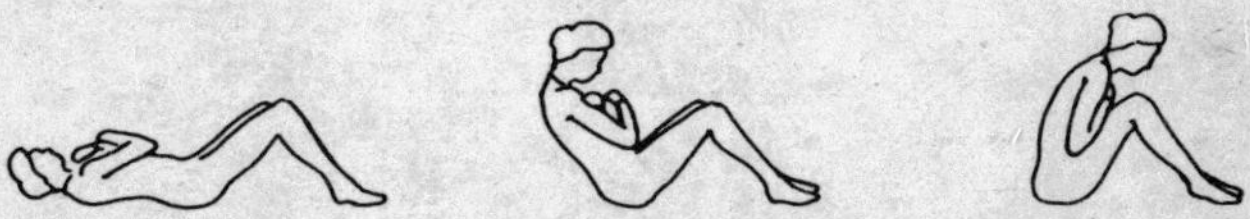

Basic Situp

Lie on back with legs well bent and arms crossed on your chest. Curl up to the sitting position and return. Do as many as are comfortable. If you cannot manage this situp, put your arms down straight at your side instead of crossed on chest.

Be sure to keep your knees bent at all times. Situps with legs straight can harm your lower back.

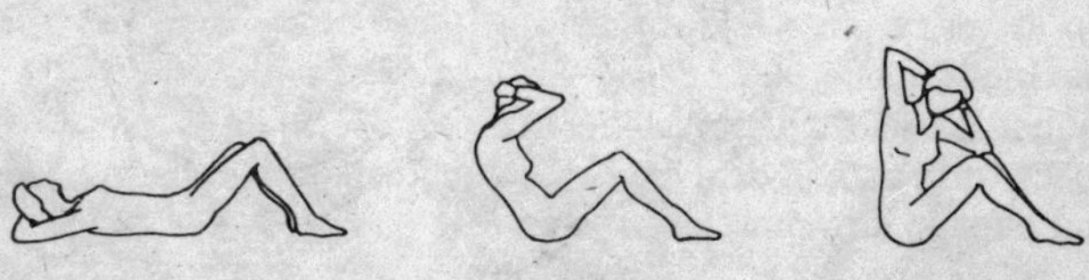

ADVANCED SITUP

A more advanced situp is done with the hands clasped behind the head. Curl up and touch left elbow to right knee (or get as close as you can). Then do reverse exercise—right elbow to left knee. The diagonal motions are good for certain specific abdominal muscles. And the position of the arms puts more stress on the abdomen than the arms-crossed position.
Do as many situps as you feel like.

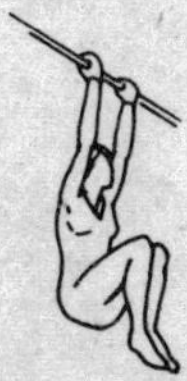

BASKET HANG

This is an excellent and simple abdominal exercise. But it requires a bar. Hang from the bar and raise your knees in front of you as far as you can. Return to starting position and repeat as often as you please.
Note: There are good expandable bars that you can install at home if you have some place they will fit, such as a high doorjamb.

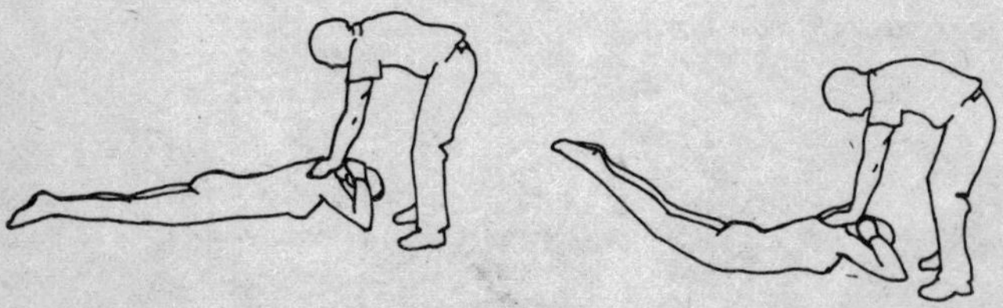

LEG LIFT (Do NOT do this exercise without medical advice if you have a back problem.)

Lie face down on ground. Raise your legs slightly. Hold five seconds. Relax. Repeat up to ten times. If you don't have a partner to help you, you will probably have to anchor your upper body by holding on to the legs of a bureau, or the top of the bed if you are doing the exercise there. Strengthens lower back.

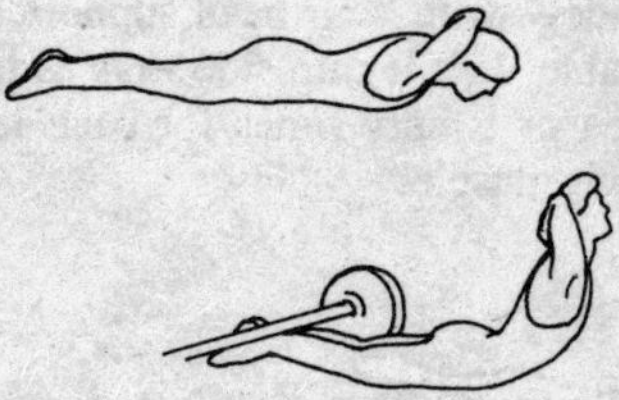

BACK LIFT (Do not overflex your back. *And if you have a back problem, do NOT do this exercise without medical advice).*

Lie face down on floor with feet anchored under a bureau—or by an obliging friend. Raise front part of your body. Hold briefly. Then lower. Repeat as comfortable. Strengthens middle and upper back.

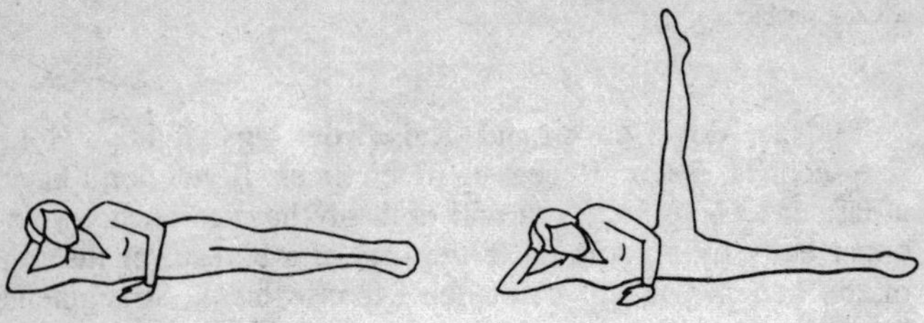

SIDE LEG LIFT

Lie on your side—with your head supported by your hand if that is comfortable. Lift leg up sideways as far as it will go. Return. Do fifteen or twenty times for each leg. Strengthens outer hip and thigh muscles.

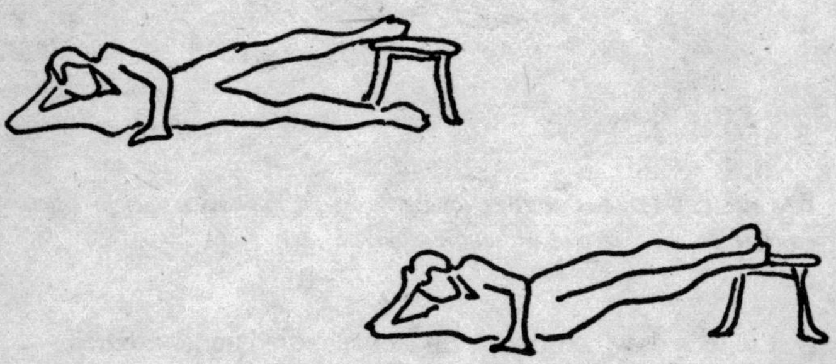

INNER LEG LIFT

Lie on left side, with your legs straight. Put your right foot on a chair, stool, or low shelf. Raise left leg up to it, then return. Do fifteen or twenty each leg. Putting weights on the ankles increases effect of exercise. Strengthens inner-thigh muscles.

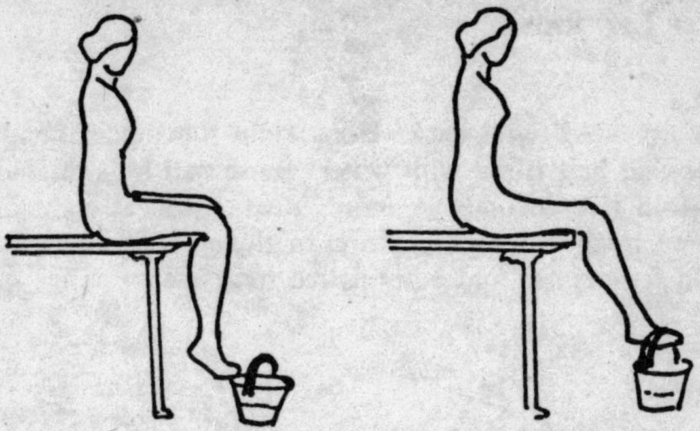

FOOT RAISE

Sit on table, well back, with lower legs hanging down. Raise a weight by flexing right foot up and holding for count of five. A plastic pail half filled with water is good if you are far enough off the ground to have clearance. Repeat eight or ten times. Then do other foot. Strengthens front muscles of lower leg. Important for runners.

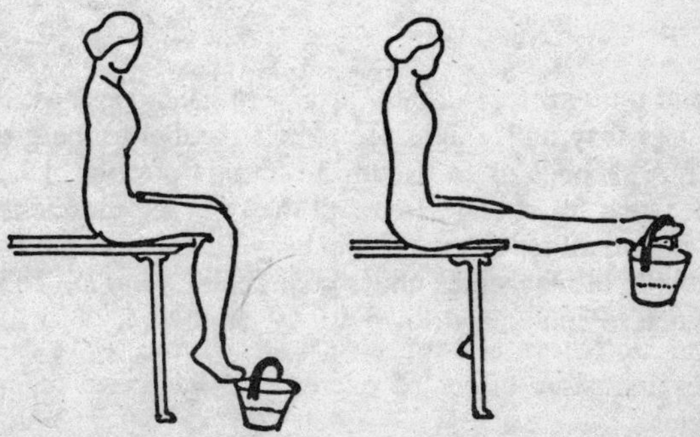

LOWER LEG RAISE

Sit on table, well back. Hook right foot under handle of plastic pail half filled with water. Raise pail by straightening leg. Hold five seconds or more. Relax. Repeat eight or ten times each leg. Strengthens front thigh and knee muscles. Important for runners and other active sportsmen.

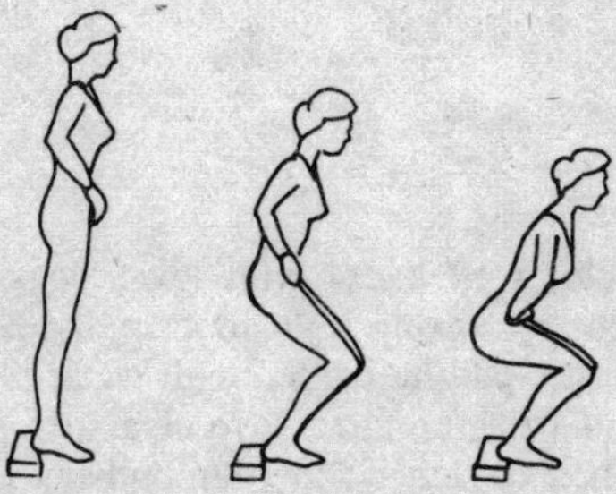

HALF SQUAT

Stand up with feet slightly apart and hands on hips. Squat down part way until thighs are almost parallel to the ground. Hold five seconds or so. Return to upright position. Do eight or ten. Great for strengthening all the front leg muscles. Specially important for skiers. If it helps your balance, put a book or a couple of magazines under your heels. *Note:* Do NOT do full squats. People used to, but they can be very bad for the knees.

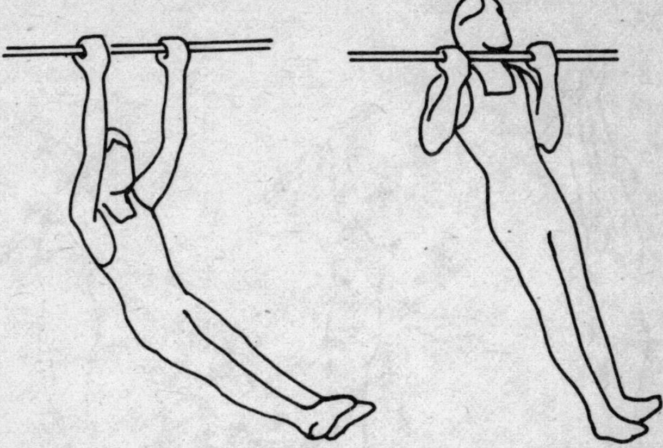

CHIN-UPS

If you have a bar, chin-ups are excellent for arm strength. Even if you can't go all the way, just trying is good. If you don't have a bar, you can do arm-curls with barbells.

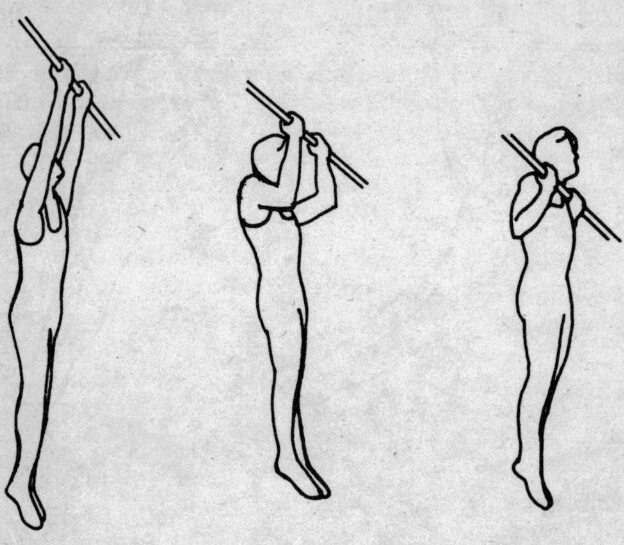

SHOULDER STRETCH

Put left hand as far up as you can behind your back, with palm out. With right arm, reach back over right shoulder, and try to touch your left hand. Hold to count of five or ten. Then reverse. Repeat several times. Stretches shoulder and arm muscles.

ENDURANCE EXERCISE

Many people don't realize there are a number of ways you can get very good endurance exercise indoors. This is important because outdoor exercise is not always practical; there may not be a good place to go in your neighborhood, or you may not have the time, or the weather may be bad. Here are some ways to get your endurance workout at home.

STATIONARY RUNNING

This can be done just about as vigorously as outdoor running. It is best not to run in exactly one spot. Move around a little. Wear good running shoes, as it is not easy on ankles, knees, and hips. If you have any trouble in these joints, choose another activity.

JUMPING ROPE

As you know, jumping rope isn't just for little girls. Boxers jump rope as part of their very strenuous training programs. If you are a novice, practice a few dozen hops first without a rope. You will also have to develop the knack of flipping the rope around rhythmically with a snapping twist of the wrist.

Ropes you buy in sports stores are good but you can also get by with a laundry cord from the hardware store. The length of the rope is important. If you take the two ends and hold them up under your arms you should be able to stand on the loop, pulled fairly snug.

Although you can in theory not do too-strenuous rope jumping at, say, 50 or 60 rope-turns a minute, rope-jumping tends to be quite strenuous. At the beginning, don't try to do more than a minute or so at a time. Slow rope-skipping is about the equivalent of a fast walk or a jog. But once you get up into the higher levels of 130 or 140 turns per minute, you are burning up something like 15 calories a minute—the equivalent of fast running.

Caution: Don't overdo. And don't jump rope if you have weak feet, ankles, knees, or hips.

Stationary Cycling

This is an excellent indoor endurance exercise.

It is easy on your joints and ligaments. If you have any problems with ankles, knees or hips, a stationary cycle is much better than stationary running or rope-skipping, which both require sound lower limbs.

You don't need to get one of the expensive stationary bikes that are all dolled up with technical wonders. One of the models under $100 is perfectly adequate.

Once you are at ease on your bike, you can supplement the vigorous leg action you get on the bicycle by giving your arms a stimultaneous workout—waving them around, raising them up and down, paddling. You can also read, knit, or watch TV.

Try keeping track of your mileage on a map—take an imaginary tour of your state.

Mini-Trampoline

Several experts report excellent results with the mini-trampoline for indoor endurance exercise. It eliminates most of the wear and tear of stationary running or rope-jumping. People who are overweight or have arthritis problems have done well with them. Some mini-trampolines come with a vertical stand which you can hold on to to keep your balance. Otherwise, you can just use it near a wall. The mini-trampoline, incidentally, is very mini. It seems to have none of the hazards of the regular-size trampoline.

Jazz Exercise

Jazz exercise—free-form moving and dancing around, either singly or in groups—is an excellent endurance activity. All you need is a good beat, enough room to move, and comfortable shoes. When done in groups, there is a leader whom everybody can follow, but there's absolutely nothing to prevent you from being your own leader at home. Or for that matter dance-exercising with whoever is there with you. As in all endurance activities, check your pulse rate a few times to see if you are in the training zone.

Stairs

Going up and down stairs can be an effective way of getting some endurance exercise indoors. Be careful not to overdo at the beginning, climbing stairs can put quite a strain on the cardiovascular system. It is best to start *slowly* and then increase your rate of ascent and descent to bring your pulse up to the training level.

Going down stairs, incidentally, is more exercise than you may realize because of the continuous braking action of the big muscles in the front of the leg. It uses between a third and a half as much energy as going up.

Important caution: There have been reports of knee trouble caused by the particular angle at which the knee is stressed in stair-climbing. So don't stair-climb to excess, and stop immediately if you have any knee pain.

Now here are some brief notes about outdoor endurance exercise.

Running

Running is one of the absolutely top endurance activities. It has gotten to be such a craze, and so much has been written about it, that I don't have to say much about it here. If you have a good place to run nearby, you can get a lot of exercise in a very short time by running. It is very easy to regulate your intensity level in running—high enough to be effective, but within safe bounds.

There is a big drawback to running—it is hard on your feet, ankles, knees. Let me stress again that if you have any problem there, it's best to go for some other endurance exercise. The same is true if you are definitely overweight.

Also remember that running doesn't do much for the upper part of your body. So, if you are a runner, complement it with upper-body activity in calisthenics or other sports or both.

Be sure to do the stretching exercises for your Achilles tendon and your back-of-the-leg muscles as well as those of the groin and the lower back. And do the strengthening exercises for your front-of-the-leg and around-the-knee muscles.

Biking

Another top endurance activity—and one that gets you around the countryside provided traffic isn't too much of a hazard.

A big advantage of biking is there's no wear and tear on the joints because of the smooth, continuous motion. So if you have any joint problem that makes something like running unwise, bicycling may be just your thing.

One important point to remember: Just getting on a bicycle and peddling along in a casual unhurried way isn't going to do much for your fitness. You have to go fast enough, or go up enough hills to reach your training level. An occasional pulse-check will help you find out if you are biking strenuously enough.

Make a point, too, of doing the basic stretching exercises for your leg muscles. There are reports indicating that bicycling shortens the hamstrings in much the same way running does.

Swimming

Yet another of the top endurance activities—provided you swim vigorously and long enough. Don't just paddle around the pool or do a languid breaststroke at the seashore.

Swimming brings into play almost all the muscles of the body and gives both the upper and lower body a good workout. It works the abdominal muscles significantly, which is more than a lot of sports do. Swimming also uses the back muscles in a vigorous but safe way.

Another advantage of this activity is that you are not bearing your own weight, so it is ideal for anyone with joint problems. Similarly, people who are overweight can get excellent exercise swimming without doing any damage to their ankles or knees.

Walking

Walking, as I've made clear in the previous chapter, is an excellent aerobic exercise and one that has been unduly neglected in the United States. It doesn't require any special equipment. All you need is a good comfortable pair of shoes. Just make a point of walking at a good clip and increasing your speed a little as the days and weeks go by. And putting in a good thirty or forty minutes or a full hour.

Cross-Country Skiing

This is a marvelous endurance activity that is more appreciated in Scandinavia and Canada than it has been in the United States. You do need some equipment—but you won't be spending the kind of money you do for downhill skiing with its resorts and ski lifts and special trails. Unlike running, cross-country skiing involves the upper as well as lower body. An additional advantage is that it is free of the jolting wear and tear of running. Since you go at your own rate, cross-country skiing has a built-in safety factor. Remember, it is a very high-intensity exercise if you push yourself, so be sure to take it easy when you start out.

Skating

Skating, either ice or roller, is an excellent cardiovascular exercise. It is a little like a gliding run. It has, however, several advantages over running. It exercises the upper body more because of the strong rhythmic motions of the arms. And, also, it is not hard on the joints. There are one of two problems, though. Finding a place to skate is one of them. And if you didn't learn to skate when you were a kid you may find it a little difficult to start now. However, it's well worth a try. With adequate sidewalks, roller skates would certainly be a sensible and healthful way to get people around our cities.

Of course everything you do is exercise to some degree. To see at a glance how various activities compare in intensity, here is a chart covering some of the exercises we have been talking about and a number of other exertions, semi-exertions, or seeming non-exertions as well. It shows you the number of calories burned per minute.

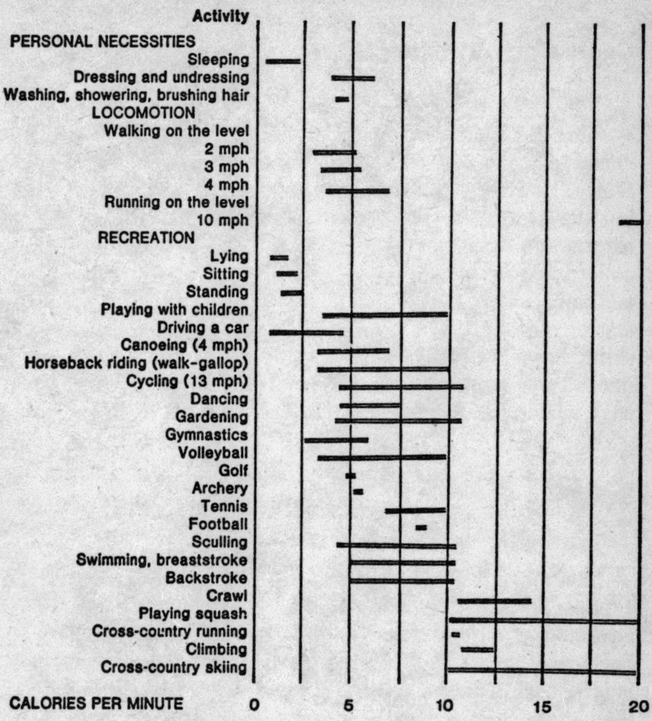

From Per-Olaf, Astrand, and Kaare Rodahl, *Textbook of Work Physiology*, New York: McGraw-Hill Book Company, 1977, appearing in "Food Facts from Rutgers."

15

Your Total High Health Plan

As I said in the preface to this book, we in the United States have now reached a point where responsibility for our health is primarily up to us as individuals. On your own, you can do more for yourself by making certain changes in your life-style than any doctor can with the most advanced drugs or the most sophisticated equipment. Bad habits can be lethal. The 1979 Surgeon General's Report on Health Promotion and Disease Prevention estimates that about half the mortality from the ten leading causes of death comes from a person's life-style. About 20 percent is due to environmental factors and another 20 percent to biological factors. Only 10 percent can be blamed on inadequate medical treatment.

Good health habits are not complicated—they are simple basics that may seem obvious to many people. This book has been about diet and exercise, which are two of the most important factors. I would like to mention very briefly some of the others, so that you can have a good overall idea of what your total health plan should be.

SMOKING

The one-sentence warning you see on a pack of cigarettes—The Surgeon General Has Determined That Cigarette Smoking Is Dangerous to Your Health—is very much an understatement. Cigarette smoking is by far the most preventable cause of sickness and death in the United States. Almost a thousand people a day—320,000 a year—die of its effects. About 10 million Americans are debilitated by chronic diseases brought about by smoking.

Smoking causes more than 80 percent of lung cancer, which is a very difficult malignancy to treat successfully. It causes cancer of the mouth, larynx, pharynx, esophagus, pancreas, and bladder. It causes chronic bronchitis and emphysema, and stomach ulcers. It is a hazard for both mother and child during pregnancy.

Although it sometimes seems as if few people are able to give up smoking, over 30 million Americans have actually done just that since the first Surgeon General's report on smoking came out in 1964. At that time, 42 percent of the adult population smoked. Today, the percentage has fallen to a little over a third. But the decline has occurred almost entirely among men. The percentage of women who smoke is just about what it was in 1964. And the most disastrous trend is that smoking among girls aged twelve to eighteen has doubled.

There is still less lung cancer among women than among men because women as a group took up smoking a good deal later than men. Rising lung cancer rates among women today reflect rising smoking rates twenty to thirty years ago. If the trend continues, lung cancer will soon become the number one cause of cancer deaths among women, taking over the lead from breast cancer.

Among my patients, I often find that long-time smokers feel the damage is done and there is not much point in giving up after, say, twenty or twenty-five years. This is not true. It is never too late to give up. Your risk of cancer and heart disease falls off very definitely after you quit.

Many young people take up smoking thinking that they can always stop after a few years. This is a dangerous illusion, as the habit—I should say the addiction—traps you quickly and can be very difficult to get rid of. The only sensible rule for smoking is If you do not smoke, do not start. If you do smoke, stop.

EXCESSIVE DRINKING

Moderate drinking, as we saw earlier, can have a beneficial effect on your cholesterol balance. And it is one of the convivial pleasures of life. But, again, I stress *moderate*. Excessive drinking is a major health risk. It can cause cirrhosis of the liver, one of the ten leading causes of death in the United States. Combined with smoking, it greatly increases the chance of cancer of the upper respiratory tract and esophagus. It plays a lethal role in traffic accidents and deaths. A pregnant woman who drinks may cause severe abnormalities in her unborn baby. And, of course, heavy drinking has an effect on a person's social and professional life.

So, if you drink, do it in moderation. Moderation in *quantity*—a sensible limit is a half bottle of wine (12 to 13 ounces) a day. The equivalent could be a couple of mixed drinks (a total of 3 ounces of whiskey or gin) or two 12-ounce cans of beer. Moderation also in *speed*—the best way to drink is when you are eating, as this slows the absorption rate of the alcohol in the blood. The worst way of drinking is to bolt a cocktail down on an empty stomach. For a pregnant woman, the best rule is not to drink at all.

CHECKUPS

Medical checkups can be of enormous importance in keeping you in good health. I am not talking here of regular examinations needed if you have a condition that is diagnosed and under treatment, but of those you should have at intervals even if you seem to be in perfectly good health.

Just what should be checked and how often depends on your age, your sex, and your personal and family medical history. Some tests should be done once a year, perhaps; others, every two, three, or five years. Few people need a so-called "complete" medical examination every year. On the other hand, as a doctor is the person who can best say what should be done in the way of tests, I think it is an excellent idea to touch base with your doctor once a year.

Of special importance are those tests which can spot serious diseases in their earliest stages, when they can be treated much more easily and effectively than they can later on. Early detection is often the difference between a passing nuisance and a life-threatening disease.

Some checks are essential for so many people that I would like to mention them briefly here.

High blood pressure affects many millions of Americans and is one of the main causes of heart disease and stroke. It rarely has any symptoms until a good deal of damage has been done. Measuring blood pressure is so simple that there is really no excuse for undetected hypertension. According to the Surgeon General's 1979 report, *Healthy People*, adults should have a screening exam for high blood pressure at least once every five years—and every two or three years if over age forty. Hypertension can almost always be easily and effectively treated with diet and exercise, or with drugs if it is on the high side. Make a point of knowing what your blood pressure is. And be sure to follow faithfully any regime that your doctor puts you on if your blood pressure is too high.

Blood cholesterol As I mentioned earlier, it is important to have a blood test that will tell you what your HDL is, and not simply what your total cholesterol is. The total reading is usually included in computerized tests that tell the doctor about a score or so of blood components, all for a fairly modest fee. A separate test for a cholesterol breakdown may be necessary, but is well worth having.

Checks for cancer are, of course, important. And the big success story here is the Pap smear, which can detect not only early cervical cancer but precancerous conditions as well. The

Surgeon Géneral's report recommends three Pap smears one year apart, starting at age twenty or at the beginning of sexual activity if it comes earlier. After that, a Pap smear every three years to age thirty-five, then every five years to age sixty, then every three years. Screening should be more frequent if a woman is on the Pill or estrogen therapy—and, of course, if any abnormalities are found.

For breast cancer, self-examination has proved to be the most effective way to detect it at an early stage. A woman should do this monthly, after the menstrual period, or on a set day of the month if she is past menopause. Any abnormality such as a lump, a puckering, or an abnormal discharge should be reported immediately to a doctor. Most often, it will turn out to be harmless, but a doctor is the person to judge.

Periodic screening by mammography is not at present recommended until after age fifty because of the very slight theoretical risk involved in the radiation. However, earlier screening may be advisable for women who are a high risk. The radiation dose of modern X-ray machines is much lower than it used to be. A woman with symptoms should not hesitate to have a mammogram on the recommendation of her doctor.

For cancer of the colon, checking the stool for occult (invisible) blood is an easy and very useful test that should be done every year or two among older adults. Periodic screening with a proctosigmoidoscope (a tube inserted in the lower bowel) is also recommended after age forty.

Everyone should be aware of the American Cancer Society's seven signs that may indicate cancer—and that should be checked with a doctor. Besides the breast symptoms mentioned above, the remaining six are:

- changes in bowel or bladder habits,
- a sore that does not heal,
- unusual bleeding or discharge,
- difficulty swallowing,
- change in a wart or a mole,
- nagging cough or hoarseness.

Eyes require periodic examinations. Of special importance is a simple test for glaucoma, an insidious disease involving excessive pressure inside the eyeball. There are rarely any symptoms until irreversible damage has been done and some peripheral vision lost. Glaucoma is effectively treated with drugs and, in some cases, surgery.

Teeth Good teeth are so important to both health and looks that everyone should make a point of cultivating good dental habits. This means avoidance of sweet snacks in between meals. It also means daily brushing and flossing. And an annual or semiannual visit to the dentist for checking of cavities and attending to them before they get too big. But cavities are actually not the main hazard for adults, especially after you reach thirty-five. Then, the main cause of tooth loss is periodontal disease, caused by deposits that erode the bone and ligament structures supporting the teeth. Flossing and brushing can help prevent this, but a professional cleaning is also needed periodically. Almost a third of the Americans between the ages of fifty-five and sixty-five have lost all their teeth. Do not become one of them.

CAR SAFETY

Car accidents are the number one cause of death among young people and the third (after stroke and cancer) for persons between twenty-five and forty-five. To say nothing of their toll of injury, disfigurement, and economic loss. Any sensible personal health plan should include some very basic, simple driving rules: drive defensively and don't speed. Don't drive if you have had a drink too many or are under the influence of a mind-altering drug. And wear your seat-and-shoulder belt. You will be doing yourself—and the country's injury and mortality statistics—a big favor.

OVERWEIGHT

Sometimes seems to be the rule rather than the exception in the United States—perhaps as much as half the population weighs more than it should. Obesity is definitely linked to at least two serious diseases, hypertension and diabetes, which can often be brought under control simply by reducing. Overweight is also associated with certain cancers (breast, endometrial, and perhaps some others as well). It is a contributing factor to wear-and-tear arthritis (osteoarthritis). So, quite aside from aesthetic considerations, you have plenty of good medical reasons to keep in trim shape.

As I have already said, the best way to lose weight is to combine diet and exercise, and not to aim at losing more than one or two pounds per week.

You can judge pretty well if you are overweight just by looking at yourself in a full-length mirror. Many people find a scale useful—if you use one, weigh yourself at the same time daily, or every other day. Tables of "normal" weights do not necessarily tell you what you as an individual should weigh. The most scientific indication is provided by skinfold measurements, at a "Y" or sports center, from which your percentage of body fat can be calculated. Good proportions to aim at are 22 or 23 percent fat for women and 14 or 15 for men.

SLEEP

The amount of sleep you need depends very much on you as an individual. Some people get along very well on five hours' a night, or even less. Some people need nine or more. For most adults, seven or eight hours is a good range. The most important piece of advice I can give you is not to start popping sleeping pills if and when you have trouble sleeping. Instead, try to find out the cause of the problem. Sleeping pills destroy the normal rhythms of dreaming and non-dreaming sleep and should be used only for special circumstances on a doctor's prescription—and almost always for only a short period. Sleeping pills have become something of a national addiction and on the average do far more harm than good.

Also, do not count on alcohol as a healthful nightcap. It may hasten the onset of sleep, but it, too, disturbs sleep patterns and causes night-time wakenings. Good sleep inducers are vigorous exercise earlier in the day, some easy activity in the evening, and a glass of warm milk just before going to bed.

STRESS AND MENTAL HEALTH

Stress is an essential part of the human condition. A life with very little stress is likely to be dull and unchallenging. However, too much stress can be very destructive. This is especially true of our modern way of living, which often puts more pressure on people than they can bear.

Often, people think of stress as psychological, but you should realize that it brings about certain definite physical changes in your body. You secrete more adrenaline. Your blood pressure and your heartbeat go up. You get keyed up to meet a difficult situation.

For our distant ancestors, this could have meant they were ready for "flight of fight," as the saying goes. But excessive stress over a period of time may be a factor in hypertension, cardiovascular disease, ulcers, and other very real physical ailments. And it can produce various kinds of mental troubles, including serious depression.

All too often, people are only vaguely aware of what kinds of things in their daily activities are unduly stressful. Take stock of just what situations get on your nerves too much—and avoid them as much as you can. Do not wear out your nerves on unimportant matters. Know your limits. Do not feel you have to be able to do everything and anything.

We also know that group support is invaluable—family, friends, church or synagogue, associations, clubs, community life. There has been a tendency to belittle the value of traditional communal institutions, but we now have a great deal of evidence showing how important they are. Modern scientific research corroborates age-old wisdom. Do not try to go it alone!

16

High Health Recipes

These recipes require preparation time. Those persons who tend to overeat need contact time with food. By spending time preparing these recipes, they did not eat so great a quantity at the meal.

Food prepared and eaten too rapidly tends to be eaten in excess.

The use of non-stick cookware is suggested for all recipes, *or* use a non-stick spray on all frying pans to avoid burning.

(*Note:* All the recipes are for one person. When you are serving more people, all you have to do is multiply each quantity by the number of people eating. It couldn't be easier, more enjoyable, or better for you!)

Research has shown that alcohol may have a beneficial effect on preventing fats in the blood from clogging your vessels. The application of this research to include alcohol as an option in the diet is no doubt controversial. If you have a problem handling alcohol, you should not drink it. However, if you enjoy a glass of wine with your meal, you could have it because it has been included as an option in the diet.

High Health Vegetables

Keep some of these on hand all the time. Serve them with lunch, as a garnish. Serve them as a dip before lunch and dinner. And have them between meals whenever you feel hungry:

Celery sticks
Carrot sticks
Cucumber sticks
Green-pepper rings
Endive slices
Broccoli flowerets
Cauliflower flowerets
Cherry tomatoes
Radishes
Green-onion sticks
Mushroom caps
Zucchini slices
Turnip slices
Fennel slices
Green beans—small and whole
Kohlrabi sticks
Artichoke hearts
Watercress
Parsley sprigs
Black olives

High Health-up

½ cup orange juice
½ cup yogurt, plain
1 teaspoon soy powder
1 teaspoon wheat germ
1 egg white
PLUS:
1 teaspoon non-fat dry milk

Combine all ingredients in a blender. Blend at high speed for twenty seconds. Pour into tall, chilled glass. *Note:* There are many ways you can vary this drink. Use different fruits—whatever is in season or what you have on hand. Or try other fruit juices together with the orange juice—grape juice, pineapple juice, grapefruit juice. Or add more wheat germ. Or try buttermilk instead of yogurt. Or soy milk.

High Health Shot on the Rocks

¼ cup V-8 juice
¼ cup jellied tomato consommé
Good pinch parsley, chopped
Good pinch chives, chopped
½ teaspoon lemon juice

Mix ingredients well. Serve on the rocks in chilled glass, with twist of lemon.

High Health Cream

1 envelope non-fat dry milk (amount usually required to make 1 quart milk)
1 cup water

Sprinkle milk powder over water. Stir with fork until completely dissolved. Store in refrigerator and use as needed. *Note:* To make High Health Whipped Cream, chill bowl and beater well, and then whip cream until soft peaks form. Vanilla flavoring optional.

High Health Sugar

- ¼ cup orange rind
- ¼ cup lemon rind
- ¼ cup grapefruit rind
- ¼ cup brown sugar

Grate rinds very, very fine. Put all ingredients in jar. Cover tightly. Keep in refrigerator and use as needed.

High Health Shake

- ½ cup fruit (fresh, water-packed, or frozen, unsweetened)
- 1 cup non-fat milk (made with non-fat dry milk or nonfat fluid skim milk)
- Pinch High Health Sugar

Blend ingredients in blender. Pour into tall, chilled glass. Sprinkle with a little more sugar. Serve.
Note: Peaches, apricots, papaya, mango, strawberries, banana, and pineapple are some of the fruits you can use. Vary the drink with whatever is in season or on hand. If you choose pineapple, use canned fruit.

High Health Dash

- 1 teaspoon dry mustard
- Good pinch oregano
- Good pinch basil
- 1 clove garlic, crushed
- Good pinch allspice

Mix mustard and oregano and basil. Add crushed garlic and allspice. Mix. Cover well. Add to salad dressings and cooking oil as needed.

High Health Tea

1 cup tea
1 wedge lemon, squeezed, or wedge of orange
A little sugar (optional)

High Health Dressing

1 clove garlic, crushed (optional)
1 teaspoon onion, minced (optional)
½ teaspoon dry mustard
1 tablespoon lemon juice
2 tablespoons soy oil
Pepper, freshly grated

Mix garlic and onion. Sprinkle with mustard. Add a little lemon juice. Blend. Add more and continue blending. Add oil and pepper and blend vigorously. Use for salad greens. For one person use half portion. Cover remaining half well and store in refrigerator.

Herbs and Spices

Herbs and spices are a wonderful way to add flavor to the foods you eat . . . without adding any extra calories. Here are some tips for seasoning vegetables:

Broccoli: Caraway seed, mustard, or oregano

Brussels Sprouts: Nutmeg or sage

Cabbage: Allspice, basil, celery seed, dill, oregano, or savory

Carrots: Allspice, bay leaf, chives, dill, mace, marjoram, mint, nutmeg, tarragon, or thyme

Cauliflower: Celery seed, curry, mustard, nutmeg, oregano or tarragon

Eggplant: Allspice, basil, bay leaf, chili powder, marjoram, sage or thyme

Green Beans: Basil, bay leaf, curry, dill, marjoram, oregano, savory

Onions: Basil, caraway seed, curry, ginger, mustard, nutmeg, oregano, sage or thyme

Peas: Basil, chervil, dill, marjoram, mint, mustard, rosemary or sage

Spinach: Allspice, basil, cinnamon, dill, mace, marjoram, nutmeg, oregano, rosemary or sesame seed

Summer Squash: Basil, bay leaf, mace, marjoram, mustard or rosemary

Tomatoes: Basil, bay leaf, celery seed, curry, dill, oregano, rosemary, sage or thyme

Turnips: Allspice, caraway seed, celery seed, dill or oregano

CLAM COCKTAIL ON THE ROCKS

¼ cup clam juice
¼ cup tomato juice
1½ teaspoons lemon juice
Pinch chives, chopped
Drop or two Tabasco

Mix ingredients. Serve on the rocks in chilled glass with a twist of lemon peel.

Madrilene on the Rocks

¼ cup tomato consommé
¼ cup potato water
Pinch celery salt
Good pinch parsley, chopped
Good pinch chives, chopped
1 teaspoon lemon juice

Mix ingredients well. Serve on the rocks in chilled glass with twist of lemon.

Herbs on the Rocks

½ teaspoon chives, chopped fine
½ teaspoon parsley, chopped fine
½ teaspoon basil, chopped fine (optional)
½ cup V-3 juice
A couple of drops lemon juice
Pinch celery salt

Mix ingredients. Serve on the rocks in chilled glass with a twist of lemon.

Tomato Sour on the Rocks

¼ cup tomato juice
¼ cup sauerkraut juice
1½ teaspoons lemon juice
Pinch horseradish (optional)

Mix ingredients well. Serve on the rocks in chilled glass with twist of lemon.

Caviar Dip

1 tablespoon red caviar
1 heaping tablespoon yogurt
A little lemon juice
½ teaspoon parsley, chopped
½ teaspoon chives, chopped

Combine ingredients and mix well. Serve with High Health Vegetables.

Green Cheese

A few fresh young spinach leaves
¼ cup parsley, chopped
2 tablespoons chives, chopped
2 tablespoons celery, diced fine
¼ pound cottage cheese
A little watercress
1 small tomato

Cook spinach about a minute in a little boiling water. Drain. Chop fine. Mix with chives, parsley, celery. Blend with cheese. Chill. Serve on a bed of watercress, garnished with tomato wedges.

Avocado Yogurt

½ avocado, peeled and mashed
1 tablespoon chives, chopped
1 tablespoon parsley, chopped
1 cup High Health Yogurt Cheese

Combine avocado, chives and parsley. Add yogurt cheese. Mix well. Serve with sprinkling of more parsley.

Herb Cheese

1 cup cottage cheese
¼ cup chives, cut fine
¼ cup parsley, cut fine
1 clove garlic, crushed
1 cup High Health Yogurt Cheese
Pinch allspice

Mix all ingredients except allspice. Sprinkle with allspice.

Cottage Cheese Scramble

2 tablespoons non-fat dry milk
2 tablespoons cottage cheese
1 egg
Pepper, freshly ground
A little margarine
¼ cup parsley, chopped

Blend milk, cheese, egg and pepper. Heat slightly in margarine. Scramble. Sprinkle with parsley and serve.

Curried Cheese Dip

½ teaspoon curry powder
1 tablespoon buttermilk or yogurt
2 tablespoons cottage cheese
Pinch celery salt

Combine curry powder and buttermilk or yogurt. When well mixed, combine with cheese and celery salt. Serve with High Health Vegetables.

Tapenade Cheese Dip

1½ tablespoons cottage cheese
1 tablespoon yogurt
A few capers
1 teaspoon anchovy paste
Good pinch parsley, chopped

Using a wire whisk, mix ingredients well. Serve with High Health Vegetables.

Piquant Cheese Dip

1 tablespoon farmer cheese
1½ tablespoons yogurt
Pinch horseradish
A few capers
A drop or two lemon juice
Pepper, freshly ground

Using a wire whisk, mix ingredients well. Serve with High Health Vegetables.

Green Cheese Dip

2 heaping tablespoons High Health Yogurt Cheese
1½ tablespoons watercress leaves, chopped
1 teaspoon parsley, chopped
1 teaspoon chives, chopped
A drop or two lemon juice
Pinch celery salt

Using a wire whisk, mix ingredients well. Serve with High Health Vegetables.

Cheese Ravigote Dip

- A few drops red wine vinegar
- Pinch salt
- Pepper, freshly ground
- ½ teaspoon soy oil
- 2 tablespoons High Health Yogurt Cheese
- A few capers
- Pinch chives, chopped
- Pinch dried tarragon or dried chervil

Mix vinegar, salt, pepper. Add oil. Combine with other ingredients. Serve with High Health Vegetables.

High Health Yogurt Cheese

- 1 quart skim milk
- ½ cup non-fat dry milk powder
- 2 heaping tablespoons yogurt "starter" (plain yogurt left over from a previous batch or from a store-bought container of plain yogurt)

Combine liquid and dry milk. Heat until milk reaches boiling point. Cool until tepid. Add starter, stirring in the yogurt well so there are little chunks all through the milk. Pour into small jars and cover securely. Set in slightly warm place (a turned-off oven of a gas range gives just enough heat if pilot light is left on). Leave overnight. Remove and chill in refrigerator. (Yogurt will keep about two or three weeks if refrigerated.)
Note: To make yogurt into cheese, drain in cheesecloth-lined sieve.

Instant Minestrone

1 cup potato water, very hot
¼ cup green beans, cooked
¼ cup carrots, cooked
¼ cup peas, cooked
¼ cup potatoes, cooked
½ small onion, minced
1 garlic clove, crushed
1 teaspoon soy oil
Parmesan cheese for garnishing

Combine potato water, beans, carrots, peas, and potatoes, or any other leftover cooked vegetables you like. While reheating them, sauté onion and garlic in oil. Add to soup mixture. Serve topped with Parmesan cheese.

Eggsprout Soup

1 cup potato water
¼ cup bean sprouts
1 egg white
Pepper, freshly ground
Good pinch parsley, chopped
Good pinch chives, chopped

Heat potato water and sprouts. Stir in egg white after mixture has simmered four or five minutes. Serve with a sprinkling of parsley and chives.

High Health Soy Soup

- 1 clove garlic, crushed
- ½ small onion, chopped
- ¼ cup celery, diced fine
- 1 teaspoon soy oil
- ½ cup soybeans, canned
- 1 tomato, peeled, cut in chunks
- Some potato water, very hot
- Pepper, freshly ground
- 2 tablespoons yogurt

Mix garlic, onion and celery. Add oil and sauté lightly. Combine with soybeans and tomato and blend until smooth. Add to hot potato water. Cook gently for about eight or ten minutes. Season. Serve, topped with yogurt.

Frutta di Mare Soup

- ¼ cup celery, diced fine
- ½ carrot, cut in thin strips
- 2 cups water
- 4 clams and their juice
- 3 oysters and their juice
- Dash Worcestershire sauce
- A little margarine
- Black pepper, freshly ground
- Good pinch chives, chopped
- Good pinch parsley, chopped

Add celery and carrot to water, bring to a rapid boil. Turn down to simmer. Add clams and their juice. Add oyster juice—reserving oysters. Add Worcestershire sauce. While mixture heats, sauté oysters lightly for a minute in margarine. Add to soup. Season. Sprinkle with chopped chives and parsley. Serve.

Winter Gazpacho

2 tomatoes, peeled, cut in chunks
1 cucumber
1 green pepper, seeded, cut in chunks
⅓ cup celery, diced fine
2 or 3 green onions, chopped
1 clove garlic, crushed
½ cup parsley, chopped
Pepper, freshly ground
1 teaspoon lemon juice
1 cup potato water
1½ teaspoons soy oil
2 tablespoons parsley, chopped
2 tablespoons chives, chopped
Cucumber slices, for garnishing

Put tomatoes, cucumbers, green pepper, celery, green onions, garlic, parsley, pepper, and lemon juice in blender. Blend well. Stir into potato water. Add oil. Stir well. Pour one half mixture in soup plate. Add garnish of parsley, chives and cucumber. Keep rest in refrigerator for another day.

High Health Vegetable Soup

¼ cup green beans, cut in small dice
1 new potato, cut in small dice
1 carrot, cut in small dice
1 cup water
1 onion, chopped fine
1 tomato, peeled, seeded, cut in small chunks
1 cup potato water, boiling hot
Whole grain bread croutons for garnishing

Put beans, potato, and carrot in small amount boiling water. Cook ten minutes at slow simmer. Add all other ingredients except croutons. Cook ten minutes longer. Serve in big soup bowl and garnish with croutons.

Cool Soup

- 1 garlic clove, crushed
- 1 small onion, minced
- ½ small potato, diced
- ¼ cup celery, diced
- ¼ cup peas
- ¼ cup carrots, sliced thin
- ¾ cup potato water, boiling hot
- Pepper, freshly ground
- 2 tablespoons yogurt
- Good pinch chives, chopped
- Good pinch parsley, chopped

Combine garlic, onion, potato, celery, peas, carrots, potato water and pepper. Cook until the vegetables are done. Remove from stove. When cool, blend smooth in blender. Chill. Serve topped with yogurt, chives, parsley.

Cream of Vegetable—Tomato consommé

- ½ cup water
- ¼ cup tomato juice
- 1 packet instant vegetable broth
- ¼ cup skim milk (made with nonfat dry milk or non-fat fluid milk)

Heat ½ cup water. Add tomato juice and packet vegetable broth. Blend and bring almost to boil. Add milk. When liquid returns almost to boiling point, remove from heat and serve.

Green Yogurt Soup

- ½ cucumber, peeled, seeded, cut in chunks
- 1 teaspoon chives, chopped
- 1 teaspoon dill, chopped, or pinch dry dill
- 1 teaspoon parsley, chopped
- A few sprigs watercress, washed, stems removed
- A few basil leaves, chopped, or pinch dry basil
- 1 cup yogurt, plain
- Pepper, freshly ground
- 2 tablespoons parsley, chopped, for garnishing

Blend cucumber, chives, dill, parsley, watercress, basil, yogurt, pepper in blender. Garnish with parsley. Serve.

Herb Soup

- 1½ pints potato water
- 1½ tablespoons fresh chervil, chopped
- 1½ tablespoons fresh chives, chopped
- 1½ tablespoons parsley, chopped
- 1½ tablespoons green onion, chopped
- Pepper, freshly ground
- 3 tablespoons Madeira wine
- A little hard-cooked egg yolk
- A little curry powder

Heat potato water until warm but not boiling. Add chervil, chives, parsley, green onion, and pepper. Mix well. Just before serving, add wine. Serve half of mixture. (Keep other half for another day.) Mix the crumbled egg yolk with the curry powder and sprinkle on soup as a garnish.

High Health Broth

- 1½ cups potato water
- 1½ teaspoons semolina
- Pepper, freshly ground
- Egg
- 2 tablespoons parsley, chopped
- 2 tablespoons chives, chopped

Combine potato water and semolina in saucepan and bring to a boil, stirring constantly. Season. Turn heat down so low it barely simmers and continue to stir another couple of minutes. Quickly add egg, and beat mixture as you add it. Serve immediately, garnished with chives and parsley.

Yogurt Soup

- 1 cup yogurt, plain
- ½ cup cucumber, cut in small dice
- ¼ cup skim milk
- 1 clove garlic, crushed
- 2 tablespoons chives, chopped
- 2 tablespoons parsley, chopped
- Black pepper, freshly ground

Beat yogurt with beater. Add cucumber, milk, garlic, and mix well. Sprinkle with chives and parsley. Season. Serve in chilled bowl.

Cream of Vegetable consommé

- ½ cup water
- 1 vegetarian-style bouillon cube
- ½ cup skim milk (made with non-fat dry milk)

2 tablespoons chives, chopped
2 tablespoons parsley, chopped

Heat ½ cup water in small saucepan. Add bouillon cube. Stir until dissolved. Add milk. Heat almost to boiling point. Garnish with chives and parsley. Serve.

High Health Celery Soup

⅔ can cream of celery soup
⅔ can water
5 tablespoons non-fat dry milk
½ cup egg white, beaten stiff
2 tablespoons parsley, chopped

Combine soup and water in small saucepan. Sprinkle in milk. Heat, stirring constantly, almost to the boiling point. Set aside to cool. Keep in refrigerator until ready to serve. Add egg white, folding it in so that it keeps fluffy texture—one spoonful at a time. Garnish with parsley.

Note: You can also do High Health Tomato Soup, and High Health Asparagus Soup, substituting cream of tomato soup and cream of asparagus soup. (High Health chicken, pea, mushroom, and shrimp soups are other variations.)

Pesto

1 cup fresh basil leaves, washed, drained, or
  ¼ cup dry leaves
¼ cup parsley, chopped
2 tablespoons corn or sunflower oil
1 or 2 garlic cloves, crushed
2 tablespoons walnuts, chopped fine
1 tablespoon Parmigiano cheese
Salt and pepper to taste

Blend ingredients in blender. When smooth enough to form a paste, serve over white or green noodles.

High Health Herb Sauce

- ½ cup yogurt
- ¾ pound Jarlsberg cheese, grated fine
- Pinch chives, chopped
- Pinch parsley, chopped

Mix ingredients. Cover tightly. Refrigerate until ready to use on:

- Baked potatoes
- Broiled fish
- Vegetables—green beans, peas, carrots, or mixed vegetables.

Curry Sauce For Fondue

- 2 tablespoons yogurt
- 1 tablespoon mayonnaise
- 1 teaspoon curry powder (or more to taste)

Mix yogurt and mayonnaise with curry powder, adding powder a pinch at a time.

High Health White Sauce

- 1 tablespoon margarine
- 2 tablespoons all-purpose flour
- 1 cup skim milk
- pinch salt
- A little pepper or other flavoring

Use either of the two following methods.

First Method:

1. Melt margarine in a heavy saucepan.
2. Blend in flour to make a smooth mixture. The best instrument for this is a wooden spatula with a flat edge.
3. Add milk slowly while stirring rapidly to prevent any lumping. Bring to a simmer, stirring all the time.
4. Reduce heat. Add salt and other seasoning, stirring well, and cook for about a minute more. Remove from heat.

Second method:

1. Blend flour with ¼ cup milk. Mix well.
2. Heat the rest of the milk in a heavy saucepan.
3. Add the flour and milk mixture and bring to a simmer, stirring constantly.
4. Reduce heat. Add flavorings and margarine and cook a minute longer, stirring constantly. Remove from heat.

Note: With the second method you don't have to use the margarine.

GREEN RICE

1 cup rice, cooked
A little tub margarine
2 tablespoons chives, chopped
2 tablespoons parsley, chopped
Pepper, freshly grated

Toss rice, margarine, chives and parsley together. Season. Serve.

Vegetable Garden Salad

- 1 tomato, sliced
- 2 radishes, sliced
- 1 beet, sliced thin, either canned or raw
- 1 carrot, sliced in thin strips
- ½ cucumber, sliced
- 7 or 8 spinach leaves
- ½ green pepper, sliced
- Several leaves escarole, Boston, Bibb or romaine lettuce
- High Health Dressing
- 2 tablespoons chives, chopped
- 2 tablespoons parsley, chopped

Mix all ingredients except lettuce, chives and parsley. Put in bowl with the lettuce. Add High Health Dressing. Sprinkle with chives and parsley. Serve.

High Health Scramble

- ½ small onion, chopped fine
- 1½ teaspoons margarine
- ¼ cup carrot, sliced, cooked
- ¼ cup peas, cooked
- ¼ cup mushrooms, sliced, cooked
- ¼ cup potato, cut in chunks, cooked
- ¼ cup green beans, cut in pieces, cooked
- 1 egg, slightly beaten
- 2 tablespoons parsley, chopped
- 2 tablespoons chives, chopped
- 1 heaping tablespoon yogurt

Put all cooked vegetables in a warm serving dish and set aside in a warm plate. Melt margarine in a skillet, add onion, and cook until golden. Turn heat down very low and add egg. Cook a minute or two, stirring constantly. Gently stir the cooked vegetables into the egg mixture. Continue cooking and stirring very gently until the vegetables are heated through. When hot, serve on toast, topped with yogurt.

High Health Salad

- ½ cup green beans, cut in pieces
- ½ cup green cabbage, cut in slivers
- 2 cherry tomatoes, halved
- ½ carrot, cut in skinny strips
- ¼ green pepper, cut in thin strips
- 1 radish, sliced
- ⅓ cup bean sprouts or alfalfa sprouts
- ¼ cup zucchini, sliced
- 2 tablespoons green onions, chopped
- 2 tablespoons parsley, chopped
- Escarole, chicory, or romaine lettuce
- 1½ tablespoons High Health Dressing

Note: This salad can be varied with other vegetables and greens in season or on hand—mushrooms, celery, endive, artichoke hearts, broccoli flowerets, and so on.

Tabbouli

- ¼ cup bulgur, cooked (follow package directions for cooking)
- 1 tomato, cut in wedges
- ¼ cup green onions, chopped
- ¼ cup parsley, chopped
- ¼ green pepper, cut in small dice
- 1 tablespoon mint leaves, dried, crushed
- 1 tablespoon lemon juice
- 1 tablespoon corn or sunflower oil
- Pepper, freshly ground

Mix all ingredients except lemon juice, oil and pepper. Combine those. Pour on mixture. Blend well. Serve on bed of Boston lettuce.

Ratatouille

- 1 small onion, chopped
- 1 clove garlic, crushed
- 1½ teaspoons corn or sunflower oil
- ½ cup eggplant, peeled, cut in 1-inch squares
- ½ cup zucchini, cut in 1-inch squares
- 1 green pepper, cut in strips
- Good pinch basil
- Pepper, freshly ground
- 1 tomato, peeled, cut in chunks

Cook onion in oil. When golden, add garlic, eggplant, zucchini, green pepper, pepper, and basil. Stir. Cook over low flame until vegetables are tender. Add tomato. Cook fifteen minutes longer, stirring occasionally. Serve. (If any is left over, or if you wish to make a double portion, you can serve it cold another time).

Tomato Zucchini Casserole

- 1 small zucchini
- 1 large onion, sliced thin
- 1 large tomato, sliced
- 1 clove garlic, crushed
- 1 teaspoon basil
- 1 teaspoon capers
- A little anchovy paste
- 2 tablespoons Parmesan cheese
- Pinch salt
- Black pepper, ground fresh

Place zucchini, tomato and onion in casserole dish. Add garlic, basil, capers. Dot with anchovy paste. Sprinkle with cheese. Cook uncovered in 325° oven for about half an hour, or until cheese is melted and zucchini is tender.

Eggplant Parmigiana

- 2 tablespoons oil
- 1 onion, chopped
- 1 clove garlic, crushed
- 1 small eggplant, peeled, sliced
- 2 tablespoons tomato paste
- ½ cup red wine
- Good pinch oregano
- Good pinch basil
- 2 slices mozzarella cheese
- 2 tablespoons Parmesan cheese, grated

In 1 tablespoon oil, sauté onion and garlic. Add remaining oil and eggplant slices. Sauté. Line shallow casserole with eggplant. Add tomato paste, wine, oregano, and basil. Top with mozzarella. Sprinkle with Parmesan. Bake uncovered at 325° about fifteen minutes or until cheese is melted. Serve (can be reheated and served later).

Stuffed Eggplant

- 1 baby eggplant
- 1 small onion, chopped
- 1 garlic clove, crushed
- 1½ teaspoons soy oil
- ¼ cup mushrooms, stems removed, chopped
- ¼ cup celery, diced fine
- A little tuna, waterpacked, drained
- A handful of fresh breadcrumbs

Divide eggplant in half, remove stem end, scoop out inside and reserve pulp. Bake eggplant halves, flat-side down, in a well-greased baking dish in preheated 325° oven for about twenty minutes. In the meantime, combine onion, garlic, oil, mushroom, celery, tuna and breadcrumbs and add to chopped-up pulp. Stuff two eggplant halves. Return to oven and bake another twenty minutes with medium heat.

Vegetable Loaf

- ¼ cup mushrooms, stems removed, sliced
- ¼ cup onion, chopped fine
- 1 garlic clove, crushed
- ½ cup green beans, diced fine
- ¼ cup celery, diced
- ¼ cup carrots, diced fine
- ½ cup potato, cut in small chunks
- 1 egg white
- 1 tablespoon parsley, chopped fine
- ½ cup High Health Yogurt Cheese
- 2 tablespoons wheat germ
- 2 tablespoons fresh breadcrumbs
- 2 tablespoons chives, chopped, for garnishing
- 2 tablespoons parsley, chopped, for garnishing

Combine all ingredients except garnish and shape into small loaf. Set on a piece of heavy aluminum foil. Bring sides up to hold loaf in place. Bake in medium oven about thirty-five minutes or until brown. Serve unmolded on platter and garnished with thick sprinkling of chives and parsley.

VEGETABLE PAELLA

½ tablespoon corn or sunflower oil
1 clove garlic, crushed
½ green pepper, diced
1 tomato, peeled, seeded, cut in chunks
¼ cup raw rice, cooked
A little lemon juice
Couple of tablespoons water
Pinch dry mustard
¼ cup green beans, chopped
¼ cup green peas
1 hard-cooked egg white, chopped
2 tablespoons parsley, chopped
2 tablespoons chives, chopped

Heat oil. Sauté garlic, pepper, tomato. Add rice, lemon juice, a little water. Mash mustard and add it to pan. Mix well. Add beans, peas, egg white. Cook ten minutes. Place paella pan in oven and turn heat to 450 degrees F for about five minutes. Turn off heat and keep in oven ten more minutes. Sprinkle with parsley and chives. Serve.

VEGETABLES EN BROCHETTE

1 big tomato, cut in quarters
1 Bermuda onion, cut in quarters
6 large mushroom caps
1 green pepper, cut in quarters
2 teaspoons soy oil

Put ingredients on skewer in alternating order. Brush with oil. Season with pepper. Broil in preheated broiler about ten minutes, turning often and brushing with more oil. Season with lemon. Serve with brown rice.

Salmon Sandwich

2 ounces salmon, waterpacked, drained
1 hard-cooked egg white, chopped
Pepper, freshly ground
Capers, drained
Wedge of lemon
1 tablespoon mayonnaise
2 slices dark pumpernickel bread

Combine salmon, egg white, pepper, capers. Add a squirt of lemon. Mix with mayonnaise. Place between slices of bread.

Tuniçoise Sandwich

1 cupful leftover vegetables—carrots, corn, green beans, limas, beets, peas, potato, whatever you have
2 ounces tuna, waterpacked, drained
1 hard-cooked egg white, chopped
Pepper, fine, freshly ground
1 tablespoon mayonnaise
2 very thick slices Italian whole wheat bread

Combine vegetables with tuna, egg white, pepper and mayonnaise. Scoop out center of bread. Fill with mixture (save the extra bread dough to make breadcrumbs).

Provolone Plus Sandwich

3 ounces provolone
2 or 3 slices thin Italian onion
Pepper, freshly grated (optional)
1 teaspoon unsalted margarine
2 slices light pumpernickel bread

Put the onion slices between slices of provolone; add pepper. Put between the bread, spread with margarine.

Aioli Sandwich

2 ounces leftover white fish (halibut or bass or sole), cut in small chunks
1 hard-cooked egg white, chopped
1 garlic clove, crushed
Pepper, freshly ground
1 tablespoon mayonnaise
2 slices whole grain bread

Mix fish with egg white, garlic, pepper, and mayonnaise. Spread bread with mixture.

Curried Egg Sandwich

Good pinch curry powder
Pepper, freshly grated
1 tablespoon mayonnaise
2 hard-cooked eggs, chopped
Enriched white bread

Mix together curry powder, pepper and mayonnaise. Add eggs. Spread on bread.

Shrimp and Watercress Sandwich

½ cup watercress, stems removed, chopped
¼ cup shrimp, cooked, peeled, deveined, diced
1 tablespoon yogurt
Good pinch parsley, chopped

Good pinch chives, chopped
Pinch celery salt
Pepper, freshly ground
2 slices whole grain bread

Combine ingredients. Pile on bread. Serve as an open sandwich if you like with an extra sprinkling of parsley and zest of lemon. Serve radishes on the side.

Salmon and Cucumber Sandwich

½ cup cucumber, chopped
¼ cup waterpacked salmon, drained
1 tablespoon yogurt
A little lemon juice
1 teaspoon capers, drained
2 slices whole grain bread
Green onions, chopped, for garnishing

Combine ingredients. Pile on bread. Garnish with onions. Serve as an open sandwich if you like, with watercress on the side.

Tuna and Mushroom Sandwich

½ cup mushrooms, stems removed, chopped
¼ cup tuna, waterpacked, drained
1 tablespoon yogurt
A little zest of lemon
Pepper, freshly ground
Pinch celery salt
2 slices whole grain bread

Combine ingredients. Heap on slices of bread. Serve garnished with a sprinkling of parsley, and with celery sticks and black olives on the side.

Crabmeat and Avocado Sandwich

½ cup avocado, cut in chunks
¼ cup crabmeat, cooked or canned. Fresh may be used when available.
2 tablespoons yogurt
A little lemon juice
2 slices whole grain bread
2 tablespoons parsley, chopped

Combine avocado, crabmeat, yogurt and lemon juice. Pile on slices of bread. Sprinkle thickly with parsley. Serve as an open sandwich with watercress on the side.

Lobster and Celery Sandwich

½ cup celery, diced fine
¼ cup lobster meat, in small pieces
A little yogurt
A little pimiento, chopped
2 slices whole grain bread

Combine celery, lobster, yogurt and pimiento. Pile high on slices of bread. Serve as an open sandwich with sliced tomato and green-pepper rings on the side.

Spinach and Tuna Sandwich

½ cup spinach leaves, chopped
¼ cup tuna, in small chunks
A little yogurt
A little lemon juice
Pepper, freshly ground
Pinch celery salt

2 slices whole grain bread
2 tablespoons parsley, chopped
2 tablespoons chives, chopped

Combine ingredients. Spread on bread. Garnish with parsley and chives. Serve as open sandwich, with cherry tomatoes and cucumber slices on the side.

Lobster (or Crabmeat) Curry

1 small onion, chopped
½ tablespoon corn or sunflower oil
1 teaspoon soy flour
1 ½ teaspoons curry powder—or more to taste
⅓ cup potato water
¼ pound lobster or crabmeat, defrosted (or canned)
Black pepper, freshly ground
Pinch cayenne

Cook onion in oil until soft. Mix flour and curry powder. Add, blending well. Add potato water gradually. Continue to stir mixture. When it begins to feel thick, add the lobster or crabmeat. Cover and continue cooking, over very low flame, for ten minutes. Season. Serve with green rice.

Note: Other ways to vary this dish are by substituting oysters, mussels, shrimp, scallops, or chicken. All are excellent.

Crab Chablis

1 small onion, chopped
¼ pound mushrooms, stems removed, sliced
1 tablespoon corn or sunflower oil
¼ cup dry white wine
½ cup yogurt, drained

¼ pound crabmeat, canned, or fresh, when available
Pepper, freshly ground

Combine onion and mushrooms and sauté in oil. Add wine. Simmer a few minutes. Add mixture, a drop or two at a time, to yogurt, stirring well. When combined, continue cooking over low heat for a few minutes longer. Put crabmeat in small, greased baking dish. Pour yogurt mixture over it. Season. Cook until golden.

Garlic Swordfish

⅓ pound swordfish
1 clove garlic, crushed
½ teaspoon corn or sunflower oil
A little lemon juice
Pepper, freshly ground
2 tablespoons parsley, chopped

Rub fish with garlic and oil. Broil about three or four minutes on each side. Season with pepper and a squirt of lemon juice. Sprinkle with parsley. Serve.

Filet of Sole Creole

¼ pound filet of sole
A little unsalted margarine
½ tomato, cut in small chunks
¼ green pepper, cut in small pieces
Pepper, freshly ground
A little lemon juice
2 tablespoons parsley, chopped

Put fish in a small, greased baking dish. Add the tomato, green pepper, pepper and lemon juice. Dot with margarine. Bake about twenty to twenty-five minutes in a preheated 325° oven. Sprinkle with parsley. Serve.

Scallops Tetrazzini

- 1 tablespoon margarine, melted
- 1 tablespoon soy flour
- ¼ cup potato water
- ¼ cup skim milk
- ½ cup noodles, cooked
- ½ cup scallops
- 1 or 2 mushrooms, stems removed, sliced
- 1 tablespoon Parmesan cheese
- Pepper, freshly ground

Combine margarine and flour (add flour, a little at a time), heat slowly, stirring constantly. When mixture starts to thicken, gradually add potato water and milk. Continue stirring until you feel it thickening. Put noodles in small, greased baking dish; add scallops and mushrooms. Cover with sauce. Sprinkle with cheese. Season. Bake, uncovered, in preheated 325° oven thirty minutes.

Crabmeat and Shrimp Ceviche

- ¼ pound crabmeat and 5 medium shrimp, cooked
- Juice of 1 lemon
- Juice of 1 lime
- ¼ cup dry white wine (optional)
- ¼ cup ketchup
- A few drops of Tabasco
- 1 tablespoon chives, chopped
- 2 tablespoons parsley, chopped
- 1 tomato, peeled, seeded, diced

Marinate cooked crabmeat and shrimp in lemon and lime juice four or five hours. Combine all remaining ingredients except the tomato, and 1 tablespoon parsley. Pour the sauce over the seafood. Cover. Chill in refrigerator until ready to serve. Just before serving, top with tomato and rest of parsley.

SOLE SHIOYAKI

1 small filet of sole
Salt and pepper to taste
Lettuce
Slices of orange
A little lemon juice

Place fish in greased, small baking dish and broil in preheated broiler. After four or five minutes, turn on other side and broil same length of time. Serve on lettuce covered with orange slices and lemon juice.

MUSSELS JAMBALAYA

2 small onions, chopped
1½ tablespoons margarine
1 clove garlic, chopped
¼ cup green pepper, cut in small pieces
1 small tomato, peeled, cut in chunks
½ cup mussels, cooked
Pinch chili powder
Pinch cayenne pepper
⅔ cup rice, cooked

Sauté onions in margarine. Add garlic, green pepper, tomato. Stir. When thoroughly heated, add mussels. Season. Turn mixture into small, well-greased casserole dish. Add rice. Mix well. Bake in a 350-degree-F oven until thoroughly heated. Serve.

Shrimp Pisto

- 1 tablespoon olive oil
- 5 or 6 shrimp, cooked, peeled, deveined
- ½ green pepper, seeded, cut in small chunks
- 1 small zucchini, cut in small chunks
- 1 plum tomato, peeled, cut in chunks
- 1 small onion, cut in chunks
- 1 garlic clove, crushed
- Pepper, freshly ground

Heat a little of the oil in a skillet. Heat shrimp a few minutes. Set shrimp aside. Add rest of oil, then all vegetables. Cover and simmer gently about forty-five minutes—adding the shrimp and stirring well after about half an hour. Season.

Baked Scallops

- ¼ pound bay scallops, washed, drained
- 2 or 3 mushrooms, stems removed, chopped
- 2 or 3 teaspoons parsley, chopped
- Pepper, freshly ground
- 2 tablespoons dry white wine
- 2 tablespoons parsley, chopped
- Lemon slice

Put scallops in small, greased baking dish. Top with mushrooms and parsley. Season with pepper. Add white wine. Bake ten minutes, or until done, in 400-degree-F oven. Serve with thick sprinkling parsley and lemon slice for garnishing.

Tuna Soufflé

⅔ cup whole grain breadcrumbs
2 tablespoons yogurt
2 small onions, chopped
1 egg white
1 small can tuna, waterpacked, drained
Pepper, freshly ground

Blend ingredients in blender. Pour into small, greased baking dish. Bake, uncovered, for about thirty minutes in 325° oven or until done.

Crab Cayenne

1 scant teaspoon margarine
1 scant teaspoon soy flour
¼ cup skim milk, made with nonfat dry milk or fluid nonfat milk
½ hard-cooked egg rubbed through a sieve (or whole hard-cooked white of egg)
Dash cayenne pepper
A drop or two lemon juice
Pinch paprika
1 teaspoon parsley, chopped
¼ pound crabmeat, canned
3 tablespoons breadcrumbs

Melt margarine, blend in flour, add milk and cook, stirring constantly, until mixture thickens. Stir in egg (or egg white), and cayenne, lemon juice, paprika, parsley, and crabmeat. Mix well. Turn into small, greased baking dish. Sprinkle with breadcrumbs. Bake in preheated, 325° oven about twenty-five minutes, or until done.

Tuna Croquette

2 teaspoons corn or sunflower oil
3 ounces tuna, waterpacked, drained
Breadcrumbs, preferably whole grain
1 small onion, chopped fine
Pepper, freshly ground
2 tablespoons parsley, chopped

While oil heats in skillet, work the remaining ingredients into the shape of a roly-poly croquette. Sauté croquette in the hot oil, about five minutes on each side. Drain on kitchen paper toweling. Serve.

Tuna Loaf

1 tablespoon corn or sunflower oil
1 small onion, chopped fine
1 stalk celery, diced fine
1 tomato, peeled, seeded, cut in small pieces
¼ green pepper, cut in small pieces
1 or 2 mushrooms, stems removed, sliced thin
1 7-ounce can tuna, waterpacked, drained, cut in small chunks
2 egg whites
A little ketchup
Pepper, freshly ground
½ cup breadcrumbs, preferably whole wheat

Sauté onion, celery, mushroom, tomato and green pepper for ten or fifteen minutes. Combine with tuna, egg white, ketchup and pepper. Place in small, greased loaf dish. Top with a sprinkling of breadcrumbs. Bake at 325° for about forty-five minutes. This makes about two portions. Serve one-half loaf and keep the other half to heat up another day.

Tuna à la Turque

¼ pound tuna, waterpacked, drained
Pepper, freshly ground
1 tomato, peeled, cut in chunks
1 onion, chopped fine
1 egg white
1 tablespoon wheat germ
½ cup yogurt, heated slightly
Good pinch cinnamon

Combine tuna, pepper, tomato, onion, egg white, and wheat germ. Shape into very small meatballs. Broil in preheated broiler until well done—about seven or eight minutes. Remove. Spoon yogurt over meatballs. Sprinkle with cinnamon. Serve.

Poached Sole

1 filet of sole
2 or 3 cups hot potato water, to which has been added some sprigs of parsley; an onion, quartered; half a carrot cut in chunks; 1 bay leaf, a little thyme
2 tablespoons parsley, chopped
Lemon wedge

Place fish in skillet. Add the hot broth. Simmer for about four minutes. Lift fish out very carefully with slotted spatula. Serve with garnish of parsley and lemon.

Shad Roe Limone

1 pair shad roe
1 tablespoon skim milk

1 tablespoon soy flour
1½ tablespoons soy margarine
A little lemon juice
Pepper, freshly ground
A little parsley, chopped
1 slice whole grain bread, toasted lightly

Dip roe in milk. Flour. Place in skillet with margarine. Sauté three or four minutes over low heat. Turn and cook another three or four minutes. Sprinkle with lemon. Season. Add parsley. Serve on toast.

Soft-Shelled Crab

½ teaspoon soy oil
½ tablespoon soy flour
1 soft-shelled crab
Pepper, freshly ground
2 tablespoons parsley, chopped
Lemon wedge

Heat oil in skillet. Flour crab lightly. Brown on all sides in hot oil. Season. Sprinkle with parsley and lemon juice. Serve.

Tuna Toss

1 small can tuna (6½ ounces), waterpacked, drained
3 tablespoons onion, minced
¼ cup carrot, chopped fine
¼ cup celery, diced
2 tablespoons breadcrumbs
1 teaspoon lemon juice
1 egg
¼ cup skim milk, made with non-fat dry milk
Pinch dill

Salt and pepper to taste
A little margarine

Toss ingredients together until well mixed. Turn into small, greased baking dish. Sprinkle with more breadcrumbs, if you like. Bake twenty-five to thirty minutes in a 325° oven. Serve.

Baked Flounder Filet

- 3 ounces filet of flounder
- 1 tablespoon onion, chopped
- 1 tablespoon tomato juice
- 1 tablespoon non-fat dry milk

Heat oven to 400-degrees F. Place fish in small, greased baking dish. Combine onion, tomato juice, dry milk and 2 tablespoons water to make a sauce. Pour over fish. Bake twelve to fifteen minutes, or until golden. Serve.

Spaghetti di Mare

- ¼ pound halibut
- 1 clove garlic, crushed
- 1½ teaspoons parsley, chopped
- 1 egg white, lightly beaten
- Pepper, freshly ground
- 2 tablespoons Parmigiano cheese
- 1 cup tomatoes, peeled, seeded, strained
- 1½ tablespoons safflower or sunflower oil
- Basil
- ¼ pound spaghetti

Chop fish in small pieces. Add a little of the garlic and parsley and blend. Add egg white, pepper, cheese. When well mixed, roll into small balls. In skillet, combine rest of garlic and parsley with the tomatoes, oil, basil. Simmer, uncovered for about twenty minutes. Add fishballs and simmer a half hour longer. Set fishballs aside in warm place. Drop spaghetti in sauce, tossing often, and cook until done. Serve with fishballs.

Fondue Indienne

1 cup potato water
1 clove garlic, crushed
Pepper, freshly ground
¼ pound shrimp, cooked, peeled, deveined, cut in small pieces
Curry sauce for Fondue

Bring potato water to a boil. Add garlic and pepper. Just a few minutes before serving, add shrimp. Serve in liquid with curry sauce on side. Serve with crusty thick slices Italian whole wheat bread.

Citrus Salmon

2 teaspoons grapefruit juice
1 teaspoon lemon juice
1 tablespoon margarine
1 tablespoon parsley, chopped
A few mushrooms, stems removed, chopped
Pepper, freshly ground
1 4-ounce salmon steak, defrosted

Combine citrus juices with margarine, parsley, and mushrooms. Season. Broil salmon five or six inches from flame for twelve to fifteen minutes. Remove. Spread with mushroom mixture. Broil two or three minutes more. Serve.

Moules Marinière

- ⅓ pound mussels
- Pot of boiling, salted water
- 1 onion, chopped fine
- 1 clove garlic, crushed
- 1 teaspoon peppercorns
- A small bunch parsley
- Pinch oregano
- ⅓ cup dry white wine
- 2 tablespoons parsley, chopped

Scrub mussels well in running water. To pot of boiling, salted water, add onion, garlic, peppercorns, oregano, parsley, and wine. Cook five minutes. Add mussels. Cover, cook ten minutes more or until shells open. Discard any that remain shut. Set mussels aside in soup dish in warm place. Strain liquid. Return to stove, bring to boil, and reduce liquid to half the amount. Place thick slice crusty French bread in bottom of soup plate. Add mussels. Pour liquid over. Serve.

Halibut in Herbs

- ⅓ pound halibut
- 2 tablespoons chives, chopped
- 2 tablespoons parsley, chopped
- A few basil leaves, chopped
- 1½ teaspoons lemon juice
- 1 tablespoon corn or sunflower oil
- Pepper, freshly ground
- 1 teaspoon breadcrumbs
- 2 tablespoons parsley, chopped, for garnishing

Put fish, chives, parsley, basil, lemon juice, and oil in bowl. Add pepper and breadcrumbs. Place in refrigerator, for a couple of hours, turning fish over from time to time. Lift fish out and drain. Grill at low heat, basting with marinade until brown. Turn over. Continue basting five minutes longer. Serve with parsley garnish.

Diced Egg with Chinese Vegetables

1 tablespoon soy margarine
1 onion, chopped
½ cup celery, diced
½ cup mushrooms, stems removed, sliced
1 hard-cooked egg white, diced
¼ cup potato water
1½ teaspoons soy sauce
1½ teaspoons cornstarch blended with water
¼ cup bean sprouts, fresh or drained canned
¼ cup bamboo shoots, fresh or drained canned
¼ cup water chestnuts
Pepper, freshly ground

Heat margarine in skillet. Add onion, celery, mushrooms. Stir fry a couple of minutes. Add egg, potato water, soy sauce and cornstarch. When mixture starts to thicken, add remaining ingredients. Stir well. Remove from heat. Serve.

Yogurt Dressing

½ cup yogurt
½ teaspoon lemon juice
1 teaspoon chives, chopped fine
1 teaspoon parsley, chopped fine
Pinch dry mustard
1 clove garlic, crushed
Pepper, fresh ground

Combine ingredients. Chill for several hours. Serve on a bed of fresh young spinach leaves or a mixed greens salad.

Fresh Citrus Dressing

1 tablespoon lemon juice
2 tablespoons corn or sunflower oil

Combine ingredients. Serve with tossed salad greens.

High Health Fruit Whip

½ cup yogurt
½ cup strawberries, cut in small chunks
Pinch grated orange rind

Combine yogurt and strawberries in blender. Blend until creamy and smooth. Serve in big bowl with sprinkling of grated orange rind.

Note: You can vary this with other fruit, such as banana or apple.

Frozen Fruit Yogurt

½ cup yogurt
6 or 7 raspberries, hulled, sliced
High Health Sugar

Chill yogurt in freezer. When very cold, beat with beater. Add berries. Beat some more. Return to freezer. When very cold, serve with more raspberries.

Note: You can vary this dish by using other kinds of fruit.

Fruit aux Fraises

1 cup strawberries, washed, hulled, halved
Good pinch High Health Sugar
1 cup orange and grapefruit sections, drained

Blend strawberries in blender. Add High Health Sugar. Pour over orange and grapefruit sections. Chill.

Macédoine of Fruit

1 California orange, peeled, sliced
1 cup grapes, halved, seeded
1 cup strawberries, hulled, halved
1 small apple, peeled, cored, cut in sections
1 small pear, peeled, cored, cut in sections
A little orange juice
A little grapefruit juice
1 or 2 tablespoons Madeira (optional)

Mix fruit in bowl. Pour in juice and wine. Chill for a couple of hours. Serve one portion (Keep the rest in refrigerator for another time).

Note: All sorts of variations are possible. Use whatever fruits are in season.

Apricot Mousse

½ cup plain yogurt
½ cup apricot halves, waterpacked, drained
Pinch High Health Sugar

Blend ingredients in blender. Blend until smooth. Chill in freezer until firm. Serve.

Apple Rosé

- 1 big red apple
- ½ tablespoon High Health Sugar
- Pinch nutmeg
- ⅓ cup vin rośe or any red diet soda

Core apple. Sprinkle with High Health Sugar and nutmeg. Pour vin rośe over it. Place in small greased baking dish. Bake in 325° oven for thirty to forty minutes. Chill. Serve.

Flurried Frost

- 2 tablespoons orange juice concentrate, semi-frozen
- 1 tablespoon grape juice concentrate, semi-frozen
- 3 teaspoons High Health Sugar
- 1 egg white
- An ice cube or two

Combine ingredients in blender. Blend well. Serve in chilled dish.

Note: Vary this recipe by using other fruit-juice-concentrate combinations.

Pear in the Pink

1 pear, peeled, cored, cut in sections
3 tablespoons vin rośe
2 or 3 cloves
Small piece cinnamon

Place pear sections in small saucepan. Add other ingredients. Heat to boiling point. Then simmer until pear is tender, basting it with liquid as it cooks. Cool in liquid. Remove spices. Serve.

Orange Orientale

1 California orange, peeled, in sections
1 tablespoon orange rind, grated
Pinch High Health Sugar

Poach orange and rind in a little water for about eight to ten minutes. Set aside to cool. Add High Health Sugar. Chill.

High Health Fruit Flip

1 cup strawberries, unsweetened, defrosted
1 egg white
½ tablespoon yogurt, plain
½ cup skim milk
A little almond extract
Pinch High Health Sugar

Combine ingredients. Blend at high speed for thirty seconds or so. Pour into tall glass. Add another pinch High Health Sugar.

Fresh Frost

1 cup canned pineapple chunks, unsweetened
A few berries—strawberries or blueberries—washed, hulled
Handful fresh mint leaves

Freeze pineapple chunks until solidly frozen. Place in blender. Blend until mixture is slightly soft. Serve immediately, topped with berries and High Health Sugar. Garnish with mint leaves.

High Health Orange

1 California orange

Peel fruit. Leave the pith on. Divide into sections. Serve.

Strawberry Snow

½ cup strawberries, frozen, unsweetened
Pinch High Health Sugar
2 teaspoons gelatin, unflavored
1 egg white, beaten stiff with 1 teaspoon lemon juice

Mash berries slightly. Combine with High Health Sugar. Cook over low heat three or four minutes. Sprinkle gelatin over 2 tablespoons cold water and add to berries, stirring until well dissolved. Chill. When mixture starts to thicken, fold in egg white. Pour into chilled bowl. Serve with topping of strawberries and High Health Sugar.

Nightfrost Grapes

½ cup Emperor grapes
A little egg white, beaten stiff
¼ cup High Health Sugar

Chill grapes and egg white. Just before serving, dip grapes in egg white. Sprinkle with High Health Sugar while still moist. Serve.

Macédoine of Melon Balls

1 cup melon balls (cantaloupe, honeydew, watermelon), unsweetened, defrosted
1 tablespoon Madeira

Put fruit in small, chilled dish. Pour wine over. Serve.

Berries in Burgundy

1 cup berries (strawberries, raspberries, boysenberries, blackberries, or a mixture), unsweetened, defrosted
2 tablespoons Burgundy wine
Good pinch High Health Sugar

Combine berries, wine and sugar. Set aside to marinate for an hour or so. Serve in chilled dish.

Tangerine Curaçao

1 tangerine, peeled, sliced, seeded
Good pinch High Health Sugar
Juice of one tangerine
A few drops lemon juice
1 teaspoon Curaçao

Sprinkle tangerine with High Health Sugar. Combine tangerine and lemon juice and pour over fruit. Chill. Just before serving, dribble Curaçao over fruit.

Strawberries and Honeydew

½ cup strawberries
½ cup honeydew chunks
Good pinch High Health Sugar
A few drops lemon juice

Slice strawberries. Combine with honeydew melon. Sprinkle with High Health Sugar and lemon juice. Chill. Serve.

Tropic Treat

½ cup mango chunks
¼ cup pineapple chunks
¼ cup papaya chunks
1 teaspoon lemon juice
A few banana slices
Good pinch High Health Sugar

Combine mango, pineapple, papaya, and lemon juice. Blend in blender five or six seconds. Chill. Serve topped with banana slices and a sprinkling of High Health Sugar.

Fruit Fluff

A few drops lemon juice
1 ice cube
1 tablespoon non-fat dry milk
½ teaspoon almond extract
Good pinch High Health Sugar
¼ cup strawberries, sliced
¼ cup pineapple chunks

Chill bowl and beater. Add lemon juice and ice cube. Add dry milk. Beat until peaks form. Add extract and High Health Sugar. Fold in fruit. Serve.

Note: You can vary this recipe with whatever other fruit is in season.

Sangria Surprise

¼ cup orange or grapefruit sections
¼ cup grapes, seeded
¼ cup pineapple chunks
¼ cup melon chunks
1 tablespoon red wine
1 teaspoon brandy
Pinch High Health Sugar

Marinate fruit in wine and brandy for an hour or so in refrigerator. Add High Health Sugar. Serve in chilled dish.

Lemon Cloud

1 tablespoon lemon juice
1 egg white, stiffly beaten
Good pinch High Health Sugar

Combine lemon and egg white, adding juice drop by drop. Beat well. Add sugar and continue beating. Freeze, stirring occasionally. Serve in chilled bowl with sprinkling High Health Sugar.

Note: A variation of this recipe is Orange, Pink Grapefruit, or Tangerine Cloud. Or for a party, combine several different kinds in one big bowl.

Coupe de Pêche

1 cup slices or chunks of peach, unsweetened, defrosted
A little peach brandy

Marinate peaches in brandy in refrigerator for several hours. Serve.

Peach Sherbet

¼ cup peach chunks, unsweetened, partially defrosted
¼ teaspoon almond extract
¼ cup non-fat dry milk powder
¼ cup ice water
Good Pinch confectioner's sugar

Combine ingredients in blender. Blend to ice-cream consistency. Serve immediately in chilled dish.

Note: This recipe can be varied with different kinds of partly defrosted unsweetened fruit.

Frullato

½ cup chilled milk
¼ cup grapes, seeded, sliced
¼ cup canned pineapple chunks
¼ cup orange sections
Good pinch High Health Sugar
Ice cubes

Combine ingredients and blend in blender until frothy. Serve immediately.

Note: You can vary this dessert with whatever fruit is in season.

Minted Blueberries

½ teaspoon lemon juice
1½ tablespoons ice-cold water
1½ tablespoons non-fat dry milk
1½ tablespoons High Health Sugar
⅓ cup blueberries
¼ cup fresh mint leaves
1 small egg white, stiffly beaten

Chill bowl and beater. Combine lemon juice and water in 1-quart mixing bowl. Sprinkle milk powder over liquid. Beat until stiff. Combine sugar, blueberries and mint. Fold mixture into whipped milk.

Fold egg white into mixture. Put in freezer. When firm, serve—topped with fresh blueberries and more mint.

Mandarin Orange in Madeira

½ cup Mandarin orange, drained
Good pinch High Health Sugar
Zest of orange peel
A few drops Madeira

Sprinkle fruit sections with sugar and zest. Add Madeira, dribbled over fruit. Chill. Serve.

INDEX

Y